ADVANCES IN

Anesthesia

Editor-in-Chief
Thomas M. McLoughlin, MD

ELSEVIER
An Imprint of Elsevier, Inc.
PHILADELPHIA LONDON TORONTO MONTREAL SYDNEY TOKYO

ADVANCES IN
Anesthesia

VOLUMES 1 THROUGH 30 (OUT OF PRINT)

VOLUME 31

Elicitation of Paresthesia, Peripheral Nerve Stimulation and Intraneural Injection: New Insight Provided by Ultrasonography, *by De Q.H. Tran, Wallaya Techasuk, and Roderick J. Finlayson*

Ecological and Economical Practice for Anesthesiologists, *by Karin L. Zuegge*

The Difficult Airway in Pediatrics, *by Jason Bryant, Senthil G. Krishna, and Joseph D. Tobias*

The Practical Management of One-Lung Ventilation, *by Wade A. Weigel and Carli D. Hoaglan*

The Role of Videolaryngoscopy in Airway Management, *by Michael Aziz*

Practical Approaches to Perioperative Blood Conservation: Acute Normovolemic Hemodilution and Antifibrinolytic Therapy in Noncardiac Surgery, *by Grete H. Porteous and Francis V. Salinas*

The Expanding Role of Multimodal Analgesia in Acute Perioperative Pain Management, *by Edward R. Mariano, Brett Miller, and Francis V. Salinas*

Advances in Perioperative and Critical Care of the Burn Patient: Anesthesia Management of Major Thermal Burn Injuries in Adults, *by Heather E. Kaiser, Cindy Meerim Kim, Sam R. Sharar, and Hernando P. Olivar*

Care of the Morbidly Obese Parturient, *by Bridget M. Marroquin*

Nanotechnology in Anesthesia and Medicine, *by D. John Doyle*

VOLUME 32

Practical Understanding of Hemostasis and Approach to the Bleeding Patient in the Operating Room, *by Albert Pierce and Jean-Francois Pittet*

VOLUME 33

The Current and Future Role of Regional Anesthesia in Enhanced Recovery After Surgery Programs for Abdominal Surgery, *by Gabriele Baldini and Francesco Carli*

Assessment and Management of Obstructive Sleep Apnea for Ambulatory Surgery, *by Rafi Avitsian and Ursula Galway*

Analgesic Techniques for Total Knee Arthroplasty, *by Lloyd Turbitt, Stephen Choi, and Colin McCartney*

Potential and Pitfalls for Big Data in Health Research, *by Karim S. Ladha, Vishal S. Arora, Richard P. Dutton, and Joseph A. Hyder*

Malignant Hyperthermia: An Update, *by Barbara W. Brandom and Patrick M. Callahan*

Current Practical Applications of Ultrasonography in Surgical Anesthesia, *by Robert A. Ratzlaff, Angela Builes, and José L. Díaz-Gómez*

Maintenance of Certification in Anesthesiology Part 4: Improvement in Medical Practice: Is It of Value and Where Do I Begin? *by Matthew D. McEvoy, Jonathan A. Niconchuk, Jesse M. Ehrenfeld, and Warren S. Sandberg*

The Prescription Opioid Abuse Crisis in America: Current Prescribing Patterns, Impact on Public Health, and the Role of the Anesthesiologist, *by Paul E. Hilliard*

Perioperative Checklists and Handoffs: Implementation and Practice, *by Aalok V. Agarwala, Suliat Nurudeen, and Alex B. Haynes*

VP Global Medical Reference: Mary E. Gatsch
Editor: Katie Pfaff
Developmental Editor: Donald Mumford

Editorial Office:
Elsevier
1600 John F. Kennedy Blvd,
Suite 1800
Philadelphia, PA 19103-2899

International Standard Serial Number: 0737-6146
International Standard Book Number-13: 978-0-323-44678-5

ADVANCES IN
Anesthesia

CONTRIBUTORS

PATRICIA J. BARR, RN, Department of Anesthesiology, Dartmouth-Hitchcock Medical Center, Lebanon, New Hampshire

JEREMY M. BENNETT, MD, Assistant Professor, Division of Cardiothoracic Anesthesiology, Vanderbilt University Medical Center, Nashville, Tennessee

JESSICA A. DARNOBID, MD, Assistant Professor, Department of Anesthesiology, HealthAlliance Hospital-UMass Memorial Health Care, Leominster, Massachusetts

NABIL M. ELKASSABANY, MD, MSCE, Assistant Professor, Department of Anesthesiology and Critical Care, Perelman School of Medicine, University of Pennsylvania, Philadelphia, Pennsylvania

VIJAYA N.R. GOTTUMUKKALA, MD, Professor, Department of Anesthesiology and Perioperative Medicine, The University of Texas MD Anderson Cancer Center, Houston, Texas

SHANNON HANCHER-HODGES, MD, Assistant Professor, Department of Anesthesiology and Perioperative Medicine, The University of Texas MD Anderson Cancer Center, Houston, Texas

NARASIMHAN JAGANNATHAN, MD, Department of Pediatric Anesthesiology, Ann & Robert H. Lurie Children's Hospital of Chicago; Associate Professor of Anesthesiology, Feinberg School of Medicine, Northwestern University, Chicago, Illinois

STEPHANIE B. JONES, MD, Vice Chair for Education and Faculty Development, Department of Anesthesia, Critical Care and Pain Medicine, Beth Israel Deaconess Medical Center; Associate Professor of Anaesthesia, Harvard Medical School, Boston, Massachusetts

JIABIN LIU, MD, PhD, Assistant Professor, Department of Anesthesiology and Critical Care, Perelman School of Medicine, University of Pennsylvania, Philadelphia, Pennsylvania

FORBES McGAIN, FANZCA, FCICM, Anaesthetist and ICU Physician, Departments of Anaesthesia and Intensive Care, Western Health, Victoria, Australia

THOMAS M. McLOUGHLIN Jr, MD, Chair, Department of Anesthesiology, Lehigh Valley Health Network, Allentown, Pennsylvania; Professor of Surgery, Division of General Anesthesiology, University of South Florida Morsani College of Medicine, Tampa, Florida

TIFFANY SUN MOON, MD, Assistant Professor, Department of Anesthesiology and Pain Management, University of Texas Southwestern Medical Center, Dallas, Texas

MARK D. NEUMAN, MD, MS, Assistant Professor, Department of Anesthesiology and Critical Care, Perelman School of Medicine, University of Pennsylvania, Philadelphia, Pennsylvania

MICHELLE C. PARRA, MD, Clinical Assistant Professor, Department of Anesthesia, University of Iowa Hospitals and Clinics, Iowa City, Iowa

BRIDGET PERRIN PULOS, MD, Instructor, Department of Anesthesiology and Critical Care, Perelman School of Medicine, University of Pennsylvania, Philadelphia, Pennsylvania

MATTHIAS L. RIESS, MD, PhD, Professor, Departments of Anesthesiology and Pharmacology, Vanderbilt University; Staff Anesthesiologist, Department of Anesthesiology, TVHS VA Medical Center, Nashville, Tennessee

MARC A. ROZNER, PhD, MD, Professor, Departments of Anesthesiology and Perioperative Medicine, and Cardiology, The University of Texas MD Anderson Cancer Center, Houston, Texas

FRANCIS V. SALINAS, MD, Staff Anesthesiologist, Physician Anesthesia Services, Inc, Swedish Medical Center; Clinical Assistant Professor, Department of Anesthesiology and Pain Medicine, University of Washington, Seattle, Washington

SURESH SANTHANAM, MD, FAAP, Anesthesiologist-in-Chief, Department of Pediatric Anesthesiology, Ann & Robert H. Lurie Children's Hospital of Chicago; Professor of Anesthesiology and Pediatrics, Feinberg School of Medicine, Northwestern University, Chicago, Illinois

JOSHUA W. SAPPENFIELD, MD, Assistant Professor, Department of Anesthesiology, University of Florida, Gainesville, Florida

AMOD SAWARDEKAR, MD, Department of Pediatric Anesthesiology, Ann & Robert H. Lurie Children's Hospital of Chicago; Assistant Professor of Anesthesiology, Feinberg School of Medicine, Northwestern University, Chicago, Illinois

PETER M. SCHULMAN, MD, Associate Professor, Department of Anesthesiology and Perioperative Medicine, Oregon Health & Science University, Portland, Oregon

JODI SHERMAN, MD, Assistant Professor, Department of Anesthesiology, Yale University, School of Medicine, New Haven, Connecticut

KARA SIEGRIST, MD, Assistant Professor, Division of Cardiothoracic Anesthesiology, Vanderbilt University Medical Center, Nashville, Tennessee

ADAM SPENCER, MD, MSc, FRCPC, Alberta Children's Hospital; Clinical Assistant Professor, University of Calgary, Calgary, Alberta, Canada

LAURENCE TORSHER, MD, Assistant Professor, Department of Anesthesiology, Mayo Clinic Rochester, Rochester, Minnesota

JONATHAN A. WILKS, MD, Assistant Professor, Department of Anesthesiology and Perioperative Medicine, The University of Texas MD Anderson Cancer Center, Houston, Texas

MARK P. YEAGER, MD, William L. Garth Professor of Anesthesiology and Medicine, Department of Anesthesiology, Dartmouth-Hitchcock Medical Center, Lebanon, New Hampshire

ADVANCES IN
Anesthesia

CONTENTS

VOLUME 34 • 2016

Advances in Anesthesia 34 (2016) xix–xx

ADVANCES IN ANESTHESIA

PREFACE

An Introduction to Advances in Anesthesia, 2016

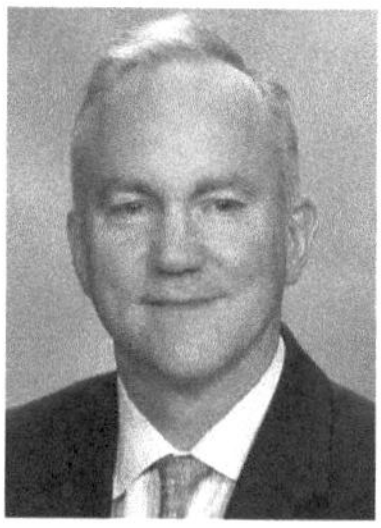

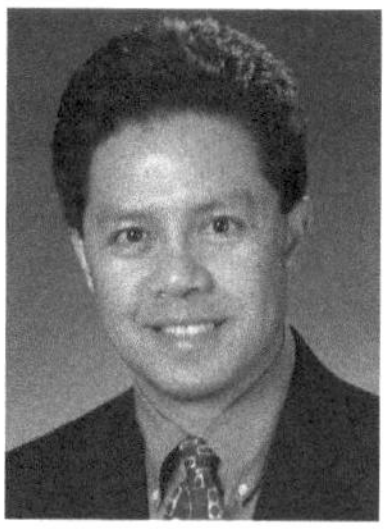

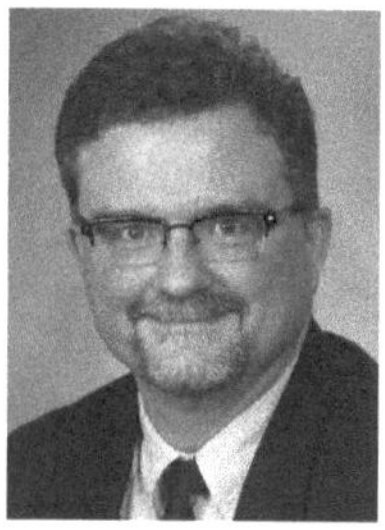

Thomas M. McLoughlin Jr, MD   Francis V. Salinas, MD   Laurence Torsher, MD
Editors

Dear Colleagues,

Welcome to the 34th annual issue of *Advances in Anesthesia*, and we thank you for your continuing support.

In planning each issue, we collaborate to identify areas of dynamic progress in anesthesiology and perioperative medicine and then to work with authors who have the expertise to communicate to our readers the context, importance, and impacts to the practice of these topics. We have different and complementary clinical interests and geographic locations, which we hope combine to bring you timely and valuable information in this issue and each year.

We apply several priorities in working with our authors. Contributions should emphasize the clinical practice of anesthesiology and thus be relevant to practicing anesthesiologists. We seek material that is timely if not forward thinking, but avoid topics of strictly academic or research interest. While other monograph-style publications often have a particular theme, we strive to provide balanced content across topics of general and specialty practices of anesthesiology and perioperative medicine. While not every issue can or does include content in all anesthesiology subspecialties, it is our editorial goal to achieve this balance over time and as we come to understand important evolution in clinical practice or changes in our understanding of the evidence bases for our anesthesia care.

As an example of the above, there are many sources for information on the organ system effects of obesity and the anesthetic considerations for bariatric and

http://dx.doi.org/10.1016/j.aan.2016.09.001
0737-6146/16/© 2016 Published by Elsevier Inc.

nonbariatric surgery. In this issue, however, you will find an excellent review of the distinctive aspects of the medical treatment modalities for obesity and the perioperative implications of drugs that are increasingly being prescribed to these patients. Another collaboration from authors across the globe from one another (New Haven, CT and Victoria, Australia) contains the thought-provoking fact that, "If the US health sector were a country itself, it would rank 13th in the world for greenhouse gas emissions," and goes on to review the environmental impact of anesthesia and to offer practical considerations to limit it. We hope that you find all eleven entries in this year's issue to honor our goals and to bring you new information that can contribute to your practice.

We welcome your feedback, to include your ideas for topics or contributors that would benefit our readers and would make *Advances in Anesthesia* even more relevant to your interests and practice improvement.

Sincerely,

Thomas M. McLoughlin Jr, MD
E-mailaddress: thomas.mcloughlin@lvhn.org

Department of Anesthesiology
Lehigh Valley Health Network
1200 South Cedar Crest Boulevard
Central Utility Building
Allentown, PA 18103, USA

Division of General Anesthesiology
University of South Florida
Morsani College of Medicine
Tampa, FL 33612, USA

Francis V. Salinas, MD
E-mail address: fvsalinasmd@gmail.com

Physician Anesthesia Services, Inc
Swedish Medical Center
Department of Anesthesiology and
Pain Medicine
University of Washington
Seattle, WA 98195, USA

Laurence Torsher, MD
E-mail address: torsher.laurence@mayo.edu

Department of Anesthesiology
Mayo Clinic Rochester
Rochester, MN 55905, USA

Advances in Anesthesia 34 (2016) 1–11

ADVANCES IN ANESTHESIA

The Perioperative Implications of New Weight Loss Drugs

Jessica A. Darnobid, MD[a], Stephanie B. Jones, MD[b,*]

[a]Department of Anesthesiology, HealthAlliance Hospital-UMass Memorial Health Care, 60 Hospital Road, Leominster, MA 01453, USA; [b]Department of Anesthesia, Critical Care and Pain Medicine, Beth Israel Deaconess Medical Center, Harvard Medical School, 330 Brookline Avenue, Boston, MA 02215, USA

Keywords

• Obesity • Weight loss • Pharmacokinetics • Lorcaserin • Phentermine • Topiramate • Naltrexone • Bupropion

Key points

- Obesity can affect pharmacokinetics, and, to a lesser extent, pharmacodynamics of administered medications.
- New weight loss drugs approved by the US Food and Drug Administration (FDA) include lorcaserin, phentermine/topiramate, and bupropion-naltrexone, each with potential implications for perioperative care.
- Lorcaserin is a serotonin 2C receptor agonist with modest weight loss efficacy and no statistically significant increase in valvulopathy. Patients on lorcaserin are at risk of serotonin syndrome. Coadministration of seritonergic agents and monoamine oxidase inhibitors should be avoided.
- Phentermine/topiramate has been correlated with the greatest sustained weight loss. Phentermine is a sympathomimetic amine and thus does have abuse potential.
- Naltrexone/bupropion is well tolerated and nonaddicting. Naltrexone is a pure opioid antagonist normally used for alcohol and opioid dependence, suppressing β-endorphin negative feedback. Bupropion may cause an increased heart rate, and blood pressure may not be reduced to the degree expected with weight loss.

INTRODUCTION: NATURE OF THE PROBLEM

According to the US Centers for Disease Control and Prevention (CDC), over one-third of US adults, or 78.6 million people, are obese, defined as a body mass index (BMI) of at least 30 kg/m^2 [1]. The Behavioral Risk Factor

Disclosures: S.B. Jones' spouse receives funds as a consultant for Allurion, Inc, which is developing a nonsurgical satiety device.

*Corresponding author. *E-mail address*: sbjones@bidmc.harvard.edu

http://dx.doi.org/10.1016/j.aan.2016.07.001

Surveillance System delineates the self-reported prevalence of obesity on a state-by-state basis. In 2014, every state had a prevalence of obesity of at least 20%; 22 states exceeded 30% or greater, and 3 states (Arkansas, Mississippi, and West Virginia) reported over 35% [2]. In 2006, the annual per capita medical spending for an obese adult was estimated to be $1429 higher than a normal weight individual, a 41.5% difference [3]. This is largely because of associated comorbidities, ranging from osteoarthritis and gall bladder disease to hypertension, coronary artery disease, obstructive sleep apnea, diabetes, stroke, and certain cancers [4].

The continuing rise in obesity prevalence can be expected to translate into a greater number of patients affected by severe obesity appearing in operating rooms and procedural suites. There has only recently been an increase in drug studies specific to or including obese patients. The US Food and Drug Administration (FDA) encourages, but does not require, inclusion of patients with obesity in most pharmaceutical trials unrelated to weight loss. Frequently, this results in insufficient numbers of higher BMI patients having been included to enable creation of specific dosing recommendations.

Obesity will influence the pharmacokinetics (PK) of a drug–what the body does to a particular medication. PK alterations may occur at several points in the system: absorption, distribution, metabolism, and/or excretion. Limited studies exist investigating obesity's effects on oral and subcutaneous drug administration. Insulin, as 1 reassuring example, shows no changes in absorption rate at equal doses in obese patients versus those of normal BMI [5].

Obesity is associated with a number of factors that can potentially affect the volume of distribution (Vd), defined as the amount of drug in the body divided by the blood concentration [6]:

- Decreased tissue perfusion
- Increased lean tissue mass
- Increased adipose tissue mass
- Increased cardiac output
- Increased splanchnic blood flow
- Changes in plasma proteins

In theory, a lipid-soluble drug has a high Vd; lipid-insoluble, low Vd. Thus, a lipid-soluble drug (as are many anesthetic medications) would require a larger bolus dose and would demonstrate a longer elimination phase. However, the nonlinear relationship between increasing adipose and increasing lean body weight at higher BMI levels [7] and the relatively poor perfusion of adipose tissue make this generalization less useful in clinical practice.

One might expect altered drug metabolism to be a significant concern, given that liver function tests are elevated in 20% to 30% of patients with obesity. However, no consistent correlation has been shown between these laboratory findings and decreased metabolism of anesthetic drugs. Conversely, phase 2 metabolism via conjugation actually increases clearance of lorazepam (glucoronidation) and intravenous acetaminophen (glucoronidation and sulfation) [8]. The final phase, excretion, is a complicated balancing act (as displayed in Fig. 1). Increased renal mass, blood flow, and glomerular filtration rate will increase renal clearance, until such time that comorbidities (eg, hypertensive nephropathy) outweigh these effects. Visceral adipose tissue may also physically compress the renal parenchyma, impairing function.

Obesity appears to less commonly affect pharmacodynamics (PD)–what the drug does to the body–independent of pharmacokinetics. For example, one study found reduced expression of adiponectin in obese mice, possibly mediating insulin resistance [9]. Drugs may exhibit exaggerated adverse effects or narrowed therapeutic windows due to associated conditions, such as increased sensitivity to the sedative and respiratory depressant effects of benzodiazepines and opioids in patients with obstructive sleep apnea. The most generalizable recommendation is to titrate to effect when specific recommendations are lacking.

Obese patients spend significant amounts of money outside of the traditional health care system. An estimated $2 billion in revenue will be generated by the weight loss service industry in 2016 [10]. Therefore, it is not surprising that pharmaceutical companies are seeking to introduce new options to promote weight loss. The FDA has recently approved several new weight loss drugs, for the first time in over a decade. These agents include lorcaserin and phentermine/topiramate, both approved in 2012, and bupropion-naltrexone, approved in 2014. A BMI greater than 30 kg/m^2 is required, or a BMI greater than 27 kg/m^2 when a medical comorbidity related to the obesity is present, such as diabetes or hypertension [11]. The 2013 American Heart Association/American College of Cardiology/The Obesity Society Guideline for the Management of Overweight and Obesity in Adults did not specifically review the evidence base for pharmacotherapy in weight loss. The authors did state, based on expert opinion, that FDA approved pharmacotherapy could be considered as "an adjunct to comprehensive lifestyle intervention" [4]. Thus, one can likely expect the increasing

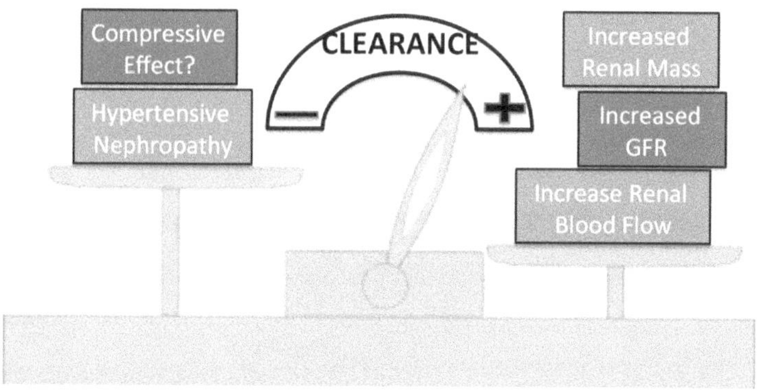

Fig. 1. The effect of obesity on drug clearance. GFR, glomerular filtration rate. (*Courtesy of* C. Ku, MD, Beth Israel Deaconess Medical Center, Boston, MA.)

prevalence of these drugs on the medication lists of patients presenting for elective and emergent surgical procedures.

THERAPEUTIC OPTIONS

Lorcaserin

Pharmacology

Lorcaserin is a selective serotonin 2C ($5\text{-}HT_{2C}$) receptor agonist. This specificity for the 2C receptor subtype is crucial, as the serotonin 2B ($5\text{-}HT_{2B}$) receptor has been implicated as the cause of cardiac valvulopathy in prior weight-loss medications removed from the market, such as fenfluramine–phentermine [12]. The $5\text{-}HT_{2B}$ receptor is mitogenic and is expressed on heart valves. Activation of these receptors leads to valve thickening and subsequent regurgitation.

Lorcaserin distributes to the cerebrospinal fluid. In the central nervous system, it activates $5\text{-}HT_{2C}$ receptors on pro-opiomelanocortin (POMC) neurons in the arcuate nucleus of the hypothalamus. POMC is cleaved into α-melanocortin stimulating hormone (α-MSH), which acts on anorexigenic melanocortin-4 receptors [13].

Lorcaserin is 70% protein bound, extensively hepatically metabolized, and 92% renally excreted. The medication has a half-life of 11 hours, and is normally dosed as 10 mg given twice daily. Lorcaserin can be taken with or without food [14].

Phentermine/topiramate

Pharmacology

The combination of phentermine and topiramate (Table 1) does not have a well-defined mechanism of action resulting in weight loss, most likely because action at multiple receptors leads to the drugs' effects. Phentermine is a sympathomimetic amine that induces anorectic effects via the release of norepinephrine in the hypothalamus, causing appetite suppression by increasing blood leptin concentration [13,15]. Topiramate increases gamma-aminobutyric acid (GABA) activity, modulates voltage-gated ion channels, inhibits excitatory glutamate receptors, and acts as a calcium anhydrase inhibitor, which inhibits lipogenesis.

Typical dosing schedules for phentermine/topiramate are shown in Table 2. As the dosage is increased, more weight loss is predictably seen, with 2% more

Table 1
Phentermine and topiramate pharmacology

Phentermine	Topiramate
(Peak plasma) 6 h	(Peak plasma) 9 h
17.5% protein bound	15%–41% protein bound
Induces CYP3A4	Induces CYP3A4
t1/2 20 h	t1/2 ~20 h
Excretion 70%–80% urine as unchanged drug	Excretion 70% urine as unchanged drug

Table 2
Typical dosing schedules phentermine/topiramate

Dosing phentermine/topiramate for weight loss indication	
Phentermine	Topiramate
Starting dose = 3.75 mg Recommended dose = 7.5 mg Full dose = 15 mg	Starting dose = 23 mg Recommended dose = 46 mg Full dose = 92 mg

weight loss in the recommended dosing versus the starting dose. By virtue of using the drugs in combination, these are lower doses of topiramate than are normally used for prophylaxis of migraines or seizures [16].

Naltrexone/bupropion

Pharmacology

Another combination drug, naltrexone/bupropion (Table 3), is gaining popularity quickly as a weight loss adjunct, due to its favorable adverse effect profile and lack of abuse potential. Bupropion has been known to cause weight loss on its own by weakly inhibiting norepinephrine and dopamine, and by stimulating POMC production. As described earlier for lorcaserin, POMC is cleaved to α-MSH and leads to decreased food intake. This precursor molecule also leads to β-endorphin production, however, which creates a negative feedback loop. This is why weight loss effects with bupropion are rapidly extinguished when it is used as monotherapy for major depressive disorder and/or smoking cessation.

Naltrexone is a pure opioid antagonist normally used for alcohol and opioid dependence. It is an important addition for augmenting weight loss, as it suppresses β-endorphin negative feedback. Use of these drugs in combination may also modify the dopamine reward pathway of the mesolimbic system [17].

Naltrexone/bupropion is typically dosed on an escalating dose schedule, as outlined in Table 4, with the maintenance dose being reached in week 4. Conservative dosing is naltrexone 4 mg- bupropion 90 mg.

CLINICAL OUTCOMES

In order for a medication to be approved for weight loss, it must be associated with at least a 5% weight loss difference between the treatment and placebo

Table 3
Naltrexone/bupropion pharmacology

Bupropion	Naltrexone
84% protein bound Hepatically metabolized Excreted 87% urine, 10% feces	21% protein bound Hepatically metabolized Renally excreted

Table 4
Dosing schedule naltrexone/buproprion

Dosing naltrexone/bupropion for weight loss indication	
Escalating dose schedule: naltrexone 8 mg—bupropion 90 mg	
Week 1	1 tablet every morning
Week 2	1 tablet twice daily
Week 3	2 tablets every morning, 1 tablet every night
Week 4	2 tablets twice daily

groups. Alternatively, a medication may be approved for medical weight loss therapy if the percent of subjects in the treatment group who lost greater than or equal to 5% of their body weight is approximately double those in the placebo group. The differences must be statistically significant. This second qualifying standard supported FDA approval for lorcaserin, the medication showing the most modest weight loss of those discussed here. Phentermine/topiramate shows the greatest weight loss potential, with weight loss being sustained even after 108 weeks of therapy as shown in the SEQUEL trial (two-year sustained weight loss and metabolic benefits with controlled-release phentermine/topiramate in obese and overweight adults). Naltrexone/bupropion is associated with middle-of-the-road weight loss efficacy, but it is a popular choice for weight modification given its lack of abuse potential. Lorcaserin and phentermine/topiramate are both classified as schedule IV drugs [18–24] (Table 5).

COMPLICATIONS AND CONCERNS

Lorcaserin

Adverse effects

The most serious adverse effect associated with use of lorcaserin is serotonin syndrome. Seritonergic agents and monoamine oxidase inhibitors (MAOIs) should be avoided in patients on lorcaserin [25]. Lorcaserin inhibits cytochrome P450 CYP2D6 and may increase codeine effects, as well as the bradycardiac effects of β-blockers metabolized via the same enzyme such as metoprolol and propranolol (Box 1). In practice, however, lorcaserin is metabolized via multiple pathways, and thus serotonin syndrome (not increased drug effect) remains the principle concern regarding medication interactions.

Although lorcaserin is 100 times more specific for the 5-HT_{2C} receptor than the 5-HT_{2B} receptor, much attention has understandably been paid to the possibility of valvulopathy with this medication. Postmarketing studies are ongoing, but phase II studies have shown no effect on heart valves or pulmonary artery pressures. A rigorous meta-analysis failed to show new valvulopathies with 1 year of use of lorcaserin. It did, however, demonstrate increases in preexisting aortic regurgitation (AR), but not mitral regurgitation (MR), in a dose-dependent fashion [26]. The ACC therefore recommends considering once-daily dosing, or avoiding lorcaserin completely, in patients with a preexisting valvular disorder, especially AR. This finding is consistent with phase III trials that studied

Table 5
Clinical outcomes of obesity medications

	Study	Results				Additional parameters improved	Addiction potential
		% weight loss		≥5% weight loss			
		Rx	P	Rx	P		
Lorcaserin	BLOOM/BLOSSUM	−5.8	−2.5	47.1	22.6	Lipid profile, glycemic control, QoL, VS	Euphoria, Hallucinations
Phentermine/topiramate	EQUIP	−10.9	−1.6	—	—	Fasting glucose, lipid profile, change in depressive symptoms, decreased waist circumference, decreased blood pressure	Amphetamine-like effects
	CONQUER	−9.8	−1.2	—	—		
	SEQUEL	−10.5	−1.8	—	—		
Naltrexone/bupropion	COR-I	−5.4	−1.3	42.0	17.0	Cardiometabolic risk markers, QoL, glycemic control	None
	COR-II	−6.4	−1.2	55.6	17.5		
	COR-DM	−3.7	−1.7	36.0	18.0		
	COR-BMOD	−8.1	−4.9	57.0	43.0		

Pooled data shown for BLOOM/BLOSSUM trials.
Full dose (15 mg/92 mg) data shown for CONQUER & SEQUEL trials.
Abbreviations: P, placebo group; QoL, quality of life; Rx, treatment group; VS, vital signs.
Data from Refs [18–24].

Box 1: Lorcaserin drug interactions

- Cocaine
- SSRIs/SNRIs
- Isoniazid
- Linezolid
- Meperidine
- Tramadol
- Trazodone
- Codeine

Abbreviations: SNRI, serotonin–norepinephrine reuptake inhibitors; SSRI, selective serotonin reuptake inhibitor.

echocardiographic examinations in 5200 patients, and found no statistically significant increase in valvulopathy with lorcaserin compared with placebo [27].

Phentermine/topiramate

Adverse effects

Phentermine/topiramate is generally well tolerated, with adverse reactions only seen if the drug is abruptly discontinued. In 2 56-week randomized controlled trials, treated patients did not have more adverse events than those receiving placebo, except in the 1% of patients receiving the highest dose range (phentermine 15 mg/topiramate 92 mg), who suffered increased incidence of nephrolithiasis.

Reported adverse effects from phentermine/topiramate are listed in Table 6. Of note, dysgusia, or altered taste sensation, results from the calcium anhydrase inhibitory effects of topiramate. Topiramate is also implicated in the central nervous system (CNS) adverse effect profile of this medication, which is why topiramate is not used as monotherapy for weight loss [20]. When used in combination, patients on phentermine/topiramate do not show increased suicidal ideation.

Naltrexone/bupropion

Adverse effects

Naltrexone/bupropion is a well-tolerated combination drug, with most adverse effects, which tend to be self-limited, occurring during the dose escalation period. Importantly, when used in combination, these drugs do not cause worsened anxiety, depression, or suicidal ideation, as can be seen on bupropion monotherapy. Bupropion can cause increased heart rate. The naltrexone component is implicated in increased blood pressure during stress, insomnia, and headaches. In combination, the most common adverse effect of naltrexone/bupropion is nausea. Also seen are vomiting, dizziness, constipation, dry mouth, and diarrhea [28]. Less common effects are tremor, hot flush, tinnitus, upper abdominal pain, and hyperhidrosis. Cholecystitis and cholelithiasis are serious adverse events reported on this medication. Naltrexone/bupropion should be used with caution in patients with renal disease, and the medication is contraindicated in patients with severe hepatic disease (Table 7).

Table 6
Adverse effects of phentermine/topiramate

CNS	Seizure, headache, insomnia, cognitive impairment, dizziness, mood disorders, suicidal ideation
ENT	Acute myopia, blurred vision, eye pain, secondary angle closure glaucoma
CV	Tachycardia, hypotension, palpitations
GI	Hepatotoxicity, dysgeusia, constipation, dry mouth
GU	↑ creatinine, kidney stones
Derm	Erythema multiforme, Stevens-Johnson Syndrome, toxic epidermal necrolysis, alopecia, oligohydrosis
Endo	Hypoglycemia
Metabolic	Metabolic acidosis, hypokalemia
Neuro	Paresthesia
Misc	Hyperthermia

Table 7
Naltrexone/bupropion contraindications and interactions

Contraindications	Interactions
• Uncontrolled hypertension • Naltrexone: patients on opioid analgesics • Pregnancy • Severe hepatic disease	Through CYP2D6 inhibition: • SSRIs • TCAs • Metoprolol • MAOIs

Abbreviations: MAOI, monoamine oxidase inhibitor; SSRI, selective serotonin reuptake inhibitor; TCA, tricyclic antidepressant.

An important consideration in patients taking naltrexone/bupropion for medical weight loss therapy is that blood pressure is not reduced as much as would be expected with a 5 kg weight loss [29]. Placebo groups saw enhanced improvement in systolic blood pressure and heart rate compared with treatment groups in studies. Importantly, diurnal variation of blood pressure is maintained, which is an important cardiovascular risk factor. However, ongoing studies continue to address the issue of whether a drug that negates cardiovascular benefits of weight loss, despite causing weight loss, is ultimately a helpful therapeutic agent. For this reason, discontinuation of this medication should be considered in patients who do not lose more than 5% of their body weight in 4 months, or in those who have a sustained increase in blood pressure or heart rate.

SUMMARY

As an increasing number of patients with obesity requiring anesthesia for surgery or other invasive procedures are seen, one must understand and integrate this knowledge into our perioperative and anesthetic planning and management. Pharmacokinetics and pharmacodynamics may be affected by the altered physiology of obesity. Specific obesity-related dosing recommendations are available for a limited number of perioperative medications; for others, it is best to dose carefully and to effect.

Concurrently, the anesthesiologist must be aware of potential interactions with the patient's existing medications. Their medications may now include one of several new agents, or combinations of existing medications, recently introduced for weight loss pharmacotherapy. Lorcaserin is a serotonin 2C receptor agonist with modest weight loss efficacy. Unlike other serotonin receptor agonists, it does not cause a statistically significant increase in valvulopathy. However, the risk of serotonin syndrome should be understood. Phentermine/topiramate is generally well tolerated, but has addiction potential because of its amphetamine-like effects. Naltrexone/bupropion has a generally favorable adverse effect profile, but is contraindicated in patients with uncontrolled hypertension and severe hepatic disease. It also presents challenges to traditional opiate-based perioperative pain management techniques, given that naltrexone is an opioid antagonist.

References

[1] Adult obesity facts. Centers for Disease Control and Prevention. Available at: www.cdc.gov/obesity/data/adult.html. Accessed April 30, 2016.
[2] Obesity prevalence maps. Centers for Disease Control and Prevention. Available at: www.cdc.gov/obesity/data/prevalence-maps.html. Accessed April 30, 2016.
[3] Finkelstein EA, Trogdon JG, Cohen JW, et al. Annual medical spending attributable to obesity: payer-and service-specific estimates. Health Aff 2009;28:w822–31.
[4] Jensen MD, Ryan DH, Apovian CM, et al, for the American College of Cardiology/American Heart Association Task Force on Practice Guidelines and The Obesity Society. 2013 AHA/ACC/TOS guideline for the management of overweight and obesity in adults: a report of the American College of Cardiology/American Heart Association Task Force on Practice Guidelines and The Obesity Society. J Am Coll Cardiol 2014;63:2985–3023.
[5] Clauson PG, Linde B. Absorption of rapid-acting insulin in obese and nonobese NIDDM patients. Diabetes Care 1995;18:986–91.
[6] Jain R, Chung SM, Jain L, et al. Implications of obesity for drug therapy: limitations and challenges. Clin Pharmacol Ther 2011;91:77–89.
[7] Lemmens HJM, Ingrande JI. Pharmacology and obesity. Int Anesthesiol Clin 2013;51: 52–66.
[8] Abernethy DR, Divoll M, Greenblatt DJ, et al. Obesity, sex, and acetaminophen disposition. Clin Pharmacol Ther 1982;31:783–90.
[9] Choi JH, Banks AS, Estall JL, et al. Anti-diabetic drugs inhibit obesity-linked phosphorylation of PPARγ by Cdk5. Nature 2010;466:451–6.
[10] Weight loss services market research report, NAICS 81219a. 2016. Available at: http://www.ibisworld.com/industry/default.aspx?indid=1719&partnerid=prweb. Accessed July 2, 2016.
[11] Jeon WS, Park CY. Antiobesity pharmacotherapy for patients with type 2 diabetes: focus on long-term management. Endocrinol Metab 2014;29:410–7.
[12] Halpern B, Halpern A. Safety assessment of FDA-approved (orlistat and lorcaserin) anti-obesity medications. Expert Opin Drug Saf 2015;14:305–15.
[13] Halford JC. Pharmacology of appetite suppression: implication for the treatment of obesity. Curr Drug Targets 2001;2:353–70.
[14] Gustafson A, King C, Rey J. Lorcaserin (Belviq): a selective serotonin 5-HT_{2C} agonist in the treatment of obesity. P T 2013;38:525–30, 534.
[15] Jequier E. Leptin signaling, adiposity, and energy balance. Ann N Y Acad Sci 2002;967: 379–88.
[16] Kennett GA, Clifton PG. New Approaches to the pharmacological treatment of obesity: can they break through the efficacy barrier? Pharmacol Biochem Behav 2010;97:63–83.
[17] Yanovski SZ, Yanovski JA. Naltrexone extended-release plus bupropion extended-release for treatment of obesity. JAMA 2015;313:1213–4.
[18] Aronne L, Shanahan W, Fain R, et al. Safety and efficacy of lorcaserin: a combined analysis of the BLOOM and BLOSSOM trials. Postgrad Med 2014;126:7–18.
[19] Smith SM, Meyer M, Trinkley KE. Phentermine/topiramate for the treatment of obesity. Ann Pharmacother 2013;47:340–9.
[20] Fujioka K. Current and emerging medications for overweight or obesity in people with comorbidities. Diabetes Obes Metab 2015;17:1021–32.
[21] Makowski CT, Gwinn KM, Hurren KM, et al. Naltrexone/bupropion: an investigational combination for weight loss and maintenance. Obes Facts 2011;4:489–94.
[22] Hollander P, Gupta AK, Plodkowski R, et al. Effects of naltrexone sustained-release/bupropion sustained-release combination therapy on body weight and glycemic parameters in overweight and obese patients with type 2 diabetes. Diabetes Care 2013;36: 4022–9.

[23] Greenway FL, Fujioka K, Plodkowski RA, et al. Effect of naltrexone plus bupropion on weight loss in overweight and obese adults (COR-I): a multicentre, randomised, double-blind, placebo-controlled, phase 3 trial. Lancet 2010;376:595–605.
[24] Apovian CM, Aronne L, Rubino D, et al. A randomized, phase 3 trial of naltrexone sr/bupropion sr on weight and obesity-related risk factors (COR-II). Obesity 2013;21:935–43.
[25] Brashier DB, Sharma AK, Dahiya N, et al. Lorcaserin: A novel antiobesity drug. Postgrad Med 2014;126:7–18.
[26] Panchal HB, Patel P, Patel B, et al. Worsening of pre-existing valvulopathy with a new obesity drug lorcaserin, a selective 5-hydroxytryptamine 2C receptor agonist: a meta-analysis of randomized controlled trials. J Am Coll Cardiol 2013;61:E1542.
[27] Weissman NJ, Sanchez M, Koch GG, et al. Echocardiographic assessment of cardiac valvular regurgitation with lorcaserin from analysis of 3 phase 3 clinical trials. Circ Cardiovasc Imaging 2013;6:560–7.
[28] Verpeut JE, Bello NT. Drug safety evaluation of naltrexone/bupropion for the treatment of obesity. Expert Opin Drug Saf 2014;13:831–41.
[29] Astrup A. Is cardiometabolic risk improved by weight-loss drugs? Lancet 2010;376:567–8.

Advances in Anesthesia 34 (2016) 13–28

ADVANCES IN ANESTHESIA

Advances in Trauma Anesthesia

Joshua W. Sappenfield, MD[a,*], Tiffany Sun Moon, MD[b]

[a]Department of Anesthesiology, University of Florida, 1600 Southwest Archer Road, PO Box 100254, Gainesville, FL 32610-0254, USA; [b]Department of Anesthesiology and Pain Management, University of Texas Southwestern Medical Center, 5323 Harry Hines Boulevard, Dallas, TX 75390-9068, USA

Keywords

• Prehospital intubation • Apneic oxygenation • Coagulopathy of trauma • Hyperfibrinolysis • Damage control resuscitation

Key points

- Managing the airway in the traumatically injured differs from managing the airway in elective patients because patients with trauma present with significant risk for aspiration, possible cervical spine instability, hemodynamic instability, and/or respiratory compromise.
- Apneic oxygenation is a technique that may increase the time to hypoxia when performing laryngoscopy.
- A rapid thromboelastogram gives quicker, more accurate results on the coagulation status of a patient who is traumatically injured compared with traditionally used coagulation studies.
- An LY30 (the percentage of the decrease in amplitude 30 minutes following the maximum amplitude of a thromboelastogram tracing) greater than 3% has been shown to increase mortality in the traumatically injured and is a possible trigger for administering antifibrinolytics.
- Damage control resuscitation should be used in conjunction with damage control surgery in selected patients for the treatment and prevention of exsanguination and coagulopathy.

Disclosure: J.W. Sappenfield received a $300 honorarium for writing an article for the *Journal of Emergency Medical Services* on apneic oxygenation in 2013.

*Corresponding author. *E-mail address*: JSappenfield@anest.ufl.edu

http://dx.doi.org/10.1016/j.aan.2016.07.002
0737-6146/16/

INTRODUCTION

Trauma is the leading cause of death and disability in adults less than 44 years of age, and has become one of the leading public health concerns globally [1]. With increased focus on the traumatically injured, there has also been an increased focus on the role of anesthesiologists who care for these patients. In 2014, the American College of Surgeons issued its *Resources for Optimal Care of the Injured Patient*, which emphasized that a board-certified (or board-eligible) anesthesiologist must be available to care for traumatically injured patients at all level I and II trauma centers [2]. The report further stated that delays in the provision of anesthesia and control of the airway were quality measures that should be recorded in the hospital performance improvement and patient safety process [2]. In addition, the report stressed that a designated physician anesthesiologist should be the liaison to the institution's trauma program and participate in their performance improvement and patient safety program [2]. This sentiment was echoed at the American Society of Anesthesiologist's House of Delegates meeting in 2014, which approved that level I trauma centers should have a trauma anesthesiology director who not only fulfills the role of trauma liaison but also has some significant training or experience in caring for the traumatically injured and participates in continuing education by earning at least 12 trauma-related continuing medical education credits every three years [3].

Multiple patient care spheres involving anesthesiology are evolving and helping to refine the care of patients with trauma. In the area of airway management, controversy exists as to whether patients should be intubated in the field before being brought to the hospital. Studies are being performed involving apneic oxygenation, which has the potential to stave off hypoxia during prolonged intubation attempts in the critically injured. The understanding of the acute coagulopathy of trauma has also improved since it was first described. It is now known that the endothelium plays a significant role and that tissue hypoperfusion leads to a hyperfibrinolytic state [4]. With better understanding of traumatic coagulopathy, new therapies (including antifibrinolytics and factor concentrates) have been studied and there has been a push for laboratory value-driven therapy. However, the treatment of abnormal hemostasis is only one piece of so-called damage control resuscitation. Other goals include volume resuscitation and prevention of hypothermia, while minimizing crystalloid administration and maintaining a low normal blood pressure.

TRAUMA AIRWAY MANAGEMENT

The "Advanced Trauma Life Support" manual recommends that airway maintenance with cervical spine immobilization be the first priority for patients who have sustained life-threatening injuries [5]. Problems with the airway and respiratory management are some of the most common errors that contribute to the death of patients with trauma [6]. In one review of 2594 deaths of patients with trauma, failure to successfully intubate, secure, or protect the airway caused 16% of inpatient deaths [7]. Airway management for patients with trauma can range from simple oxygen administration for patients who are able to protect their airways to emergency tracheal intubation for patients who are obtunded, unable to maintain their airways, or hypoxic. Delays in proper airway management can lead to severe consequences, including increased mortality [8]. Furthermore, inadequate airway management can cause secondary injury such as aspiration, hypoxia, hemodynamic instability, or cervical injury [9]. The Eastern Association for the Surgery of Trauma has published practice management guidelines on emergency tracheal intubation immediately following traumatic injury (Box 1) [10].

Standard difficult airway algorithms [11] may not be applicable to patients with trauma for a variety of reasons. For patients thought to have a difficult airway because of either preexisting conditions or traumatic injuries, awake fiberoptic intubation may not be a feasible option because of lack of time or equipment, or because blood in the airway obscures adequate view. Furthermore, in acutely injured patients with trauma, it is almost never an option to awaken the patient. Unlike elective intubations, traumatic airway management is frequently accompanied by hemodynamic instability, significant risk for aspiration, cervical immobilization, and/or direct airway trauma. Trauma centers should have modified difficult airway scenarios for patients with trauma that include the use of airway adjuncts and rescue techniques [12].

All patients who have experienced significant blunt trauma should be in a cervical collar to prevent secondary injury [13]. Airway management for these patients indicates the assistance of an additional provider who can hold manual

Box 1: Level 1 indications for emergency tracheal intubation

For patients with trauma with any of the following traits:

- Airway obstruction
- Hypoventilation
- Persistent hypoxemia ($SaO_2 \leq 90\%$) despite supplemental O_2
- Severe cognitive impairment ($GCS \leq 8$)
- Severe hemorrhagic shock
- Cardiac arrest

For patients experiencing smoke inhalation with any of the following traits:

- Major burn greater than or equal to 40% of BSA
- Major burns and/or smoke inhalation with an anticipated prolonged transport time to definitive care
- Impending airway obstruction, such as moderate to severe facial burn, oropharyngeal burn, or airway injury seen on endoscopy

Abbreviations: BSA, body surface area; GCS, Glasgow Coma Scale; SaO_2, arterial oxygen saturation.

in-line stabilization. The anterior portion of a cervical collar should be removed for laryngoscopy because it can limit mouth opening and make intubation more difficult [14]. Some investigators have argued that manual in-line stabilization increases the pressure applied by the laryngoscope [15], but it continues to be the standard of care to prevent secondary neurologic injury [14]. Video laryngoscopy has become widely available over the past decade, and is an important adjunct in the airway management of patients with trauma. Many investigators have shown the benefits of various video laryngoscopes compared with direct laryngoscopy, including improved Cormack-Lehane grade [16], improved first-attempt success rates [17], decreased incidence of esophageal intubation [17], less cervical spine movement [18–20], and decreased hemodynamic responses [21]. However, others have found no attenuation in hemodynamic responses [22] or improvement in intubation times [23] with video laryngoscopes. Video laryngoscopes have shown success rates similar to those of direct laryngoscopy for patients with nondifficult airways, but may be more advantageous when airway anatomy is difficult [24–26]. At this time, there is insufficient evidence to recommend the routine use of video rather than direct laryngoscopy for emergency tracheal intubation [10].

PREHOSPITAL AIRWAY MANAGEMENT

In the United States, prehospital trauma care is usually provided by the emergency medical system, which is staffed by paramedics and emergency medical technicians [27]. Prehospital intubation has been debated by many investigators, with some citing improved outcomes in patients who are intubated before reaching the hospital [28], whereas others have shown worse outcomes [29,30]. Prehospital intubation may be beneficial for rural settings, but in cities where transportation to a trauma center is expeditious, many have argued that the scoop-and-run method can save lives and that noncritical airway intervention should not delay transport to the hospital [28,31]. At the center of these arguments is the question of who is best equipped to provide airway management to these critically ill patients while minimizing any adverse effects from induction, intubation, and positive pressure ventilation. In a busy, large, urban trauma center, a prospective study showed a 31% incidence of failed prehospital intubation performed by paramedics, with 12% of patients arriving with unrecognized esophageal intubation [32]. This finding is in stark contrast with a series of prehospital intubations in France, where senior emergency physicians were successful in 97% of intubations, suggesting that provider experience plays an important role in the success rate [33]. Similarly, Davis and colleagues [34] found that systems with more experience with intubation had lower adjusted mortality scores compared with systems that did not have as much experience with out-of-hospital intubations. A meta-analysis of prehospital intubations found that the failure rate of physician-manned prehospital teams was 1 of 100 patients, whereas nonphysicians failed an average of 15 times per 100 attempts [35]. The experience advantage not only exists between paramedics and physicians but also among physicians. Separating physicians into proficient versus expert performers based on their experience, Breckwoldt and colleagues [36] showed that expert physicians had an incidence of difficult intubation that was about one-half that of proficient performers.

Other possible hazards with prehospital intubations are the physiologic changes that accompany positive pressure ventilation. In a swine model of hemorrhagic shock, the intubated group had more hemorrhage, worse hypothermia, and higher lactate levels than the nonintubated group [37]. Thus, the investigators concluded that, for patients with penetrating trauma, prehospital intubation should be foregone in favor of immediate transportation to definitive care. In a retrospective review of emergent endotracheal intubation in patients with trauma at a large trauma center, anesthesiologists had a 99.7% success rate, showing that, once patients arrive at a trauma center, airway management is much more successful than in the field [12]. Some investigators have proposed a so-called gold, silver, and bronze strategy of airway management, depending on the individual responder's clinical experience with airway management. The gold standard comprises providers who have daily experience with, and can safely provide, prehospital intubation. The silver standard comprises less experienced providers who should use alternative supraglottic devices first. The bronze standard comprises providers with infrequent experience who should concentrate on bag-valve-mask ventilation as the primary method of airway management (Table 1) [38,39].

Studies comparing the use of supraglottic devices versus endotracheal intubation in prehospital patients with trauma have found no difference in effective ventilation or mortality [40,41]. Similarly, prehospital intubation does not seem to increase survival compared with bag-valve-mask ventilation in patients with trauma [30]. At present, no airway device is optimal for a certain type of provider or certain level of experience to ensure the safest airway management. A Cochrane Review of studies with different types of providers, patients, injuries, and airway management techniques concluded that the "skill level of the operator may be key in determining efficacy" [42]. In systems that cannot provide safe and effective prehospital endotracheal intubation, efforts should be focused on providing basic airway management and ventilation [43].

APNEIC OXYGENATION

Preoxygenation (or denitrogenation) of patients before induction and intubation is widely practiced to increase oxygen reserve, delay the onset of hypoxia,

Table 1
Proposed gold, silver, and bronze strategies for airway management

Frequency of clinical airway management experience	Color	Suggested first-line airway management technique
Daily	Gold	Prehospital tracheal intubation
Frequent (but not daily)	Silver	Supraglottic devices
Infrequent	Bronze	Bag-valve-mask ventilation

and increase the time for laryngoscopy and tracheal intubation. In addition to preoxygenation, the duration of apnea tolerated before oxyhemoglobin desaturation can also be increased with apneic oxygenation, first described by Frumin and colleagues [44] in 1959. Healthy volunteers were able to maintain 100% oxygen saturation (SpO_2) for up to 55 minutes while receiving apneic oxygenation. However, CO_2 continues to accumulate without ventilation and patients can become profoundly acidotic if ventilation is not resumed [44]. Using 6 L/min of oxygen by nasal cannula, Ramachandran and colleagues [45] showed a significant increase in the frequency and duration of SpO_2 greater than or equal to 95% and a higher minimum SpO_2 during prolonged laryngoscopy in obese patients. A recent study by Semler and colleagues [46] failed to show that apneic oxygenation increased the lowest arterial saturation during intubation compared with usual preoxygenation techniques alone in critically ill patients. The investigators concluded that patients who are critically ill with poor pulmonary function in a medical intensive care unit might not benefit as much from apneic oxygenation as those who are being electively intubated in the operating room for surgery. Rates of oxygen delivery for apneic oxygenation have ranged from 6 to 60 L/min [45–47]. The presence of the nasal cannula can cause a leak because of an imperfect mask seal (Fig. 1), but it can always be removed if it is interfering with mask ventilation. The application of apneic oxygenation can provide several more minutes to secure the airway before oxygenation is inadequate [48]. It is recommended that nasal cannula oxygen be applied in addition to standard preoxygenation in high-risk patients [49].

ACUTE COAGULOPATHY OF TRAUMA

The incidence of coagulopathy in trauma is between 24% and 34% [50–53]. Factors associated with coagulopathy include hypothermia, acidosis, dilution of coagulation factors, consumption of coagulation factors, higher base deficits,

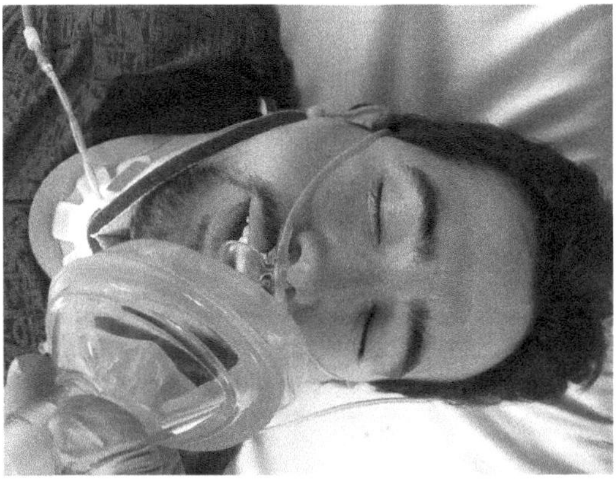

Fig. 1. Application of nasal cannula oxygen to facilitate apneic oxygenation during laryngoscopy.

hypoperfusion, greater volumes of crystalloid intravenous fluids, tissue damage, inflammation, and injury severity [51,54–60]. Although the coagulopathy of trauma has been characterized using standard hemostasis parameters, such as prothrombin time (PT) and International Normalized Ratio (INR), activated partial thromboplastin time (PTT), platelet count, and fibrinogen levels, there is evidence that these studies do not correlate well with postoperative hemorrhagic complications [61–63]. More recently, the risk of hemorrhage in patients with trauma has been evaluated by rapid thromboelastograms (TEGs) [64]. TEGs have been shown to better correlate with the need for blood product transfusions than PT, PTT, and INR [65]. Rapid TEGs are also better suited for evaluation of the degree of fibrinolytic activity. Specifically, an LY30 (the percentage of the decrease in amplitude 30 minutes following the maximum amplitude of the TEG tracing) greater than 3% is associated with an odds ratio of 4 for mortality, and a higher likelihood of massive transfusion (Fig. 2) [66,67].

The incidence of traumatically injured patients with an injury severity score greater than 15 and an LY30 greater than 3% has been reported at 18% [68]. Clinicians should be aware that the LY30 on a rapid TEG may poorly correlate with the LY30 on a standard TEG [69,70], and the significance of 3% should not be used interchangeably.

Hyperfibrinolysis observed in patients with trauma is associated with larger volumes of infused crystalloid [66] and seems to be caused by increased activated protein C, leading to increased levels of tissue plasminogen activator (tPA) [4]. Higher concentrations of circulating tPA are measured in traumatically injured patients, and the clots formed are more susceptible to being degraded by tPA [71]. In addition, Moore and colleagues [71] found that,

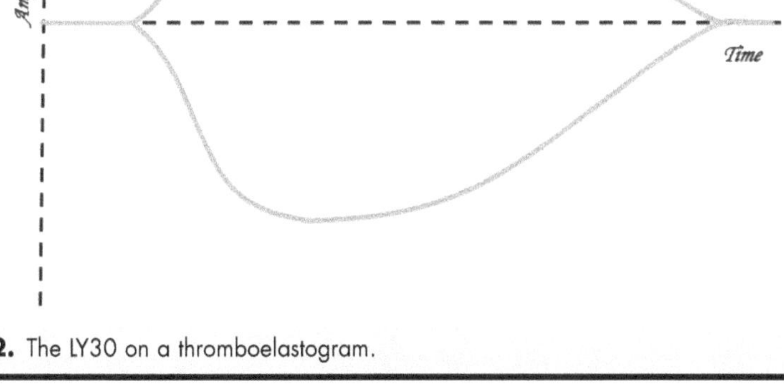

Fig. 2. The LY30 on a thromboelastogram.

although the clots that form in patients with trauma are more susceptible to fibrinolysis, these patients made quicker, stronger thrombi compared with non-injured controls. This process seems to be platelet mediated and initiated by an unknown metabolite affecting the ADP pathway [71]. Of note, when whole blood is mixed with hemolyzed cells, it similarly forms more rapid clot that is measurably stronger, but is more prone to fibrinolysis [72].

It is possible that the association between hyperfibrinolysis and coagulopathy during trauma inspired the Clinical Randomisation of an Antifibrinolytic in Significant Haemorrhage (CRASH 2) study, published in 2010 [73]. Shakur and colleagues [73] found that the administration of tranexamic acid (Cyklokapron) as a bolus followed by an infusion reduced the all-cause mortality of participants by 1.5%. Because of methodological issues with the study (eg, nonspecific inclusion criteria, absent laboratory data, infrequency of significant hemorrhage), it is difficult to apply the results to modern trauma centers. However, the significant reduction in mortality has led to wide use of the drug. For example, the use of tranexamic acid in the prehospital setting for civilians and combat casualties in Israel has been reported [74], as well as in traumatically injured children [75]. There is even a Cochrane Review showing a 30% reduction in the need for transfusion when tranexamic acid is administered for emergent surgery, but no reduction in mortality [76]. Because of the relative absence of complications related to tranexamic acid in the CRASH 2 study, guidelines for its use have ranged from the inclusion criteria of the CRASH 2 study to administration based on laboratory results [77]. Plasmin-antiplasmin complex levels seem to be more sensitive than rotational thromboelastometry at detecting hyperfibrinolysis, but clinical significance has yet to be proved [78].

There has been concern over arbitrarily administering tranexamic acid in the trauma community. Moore and colleagues [68] showed that 18% of all patients arriving acutely injured to a trauma center with an injury severity score greater than 15 had an LY30 greater than 3%. These patients were more likely to require a transfusion of any blood product, a massive transfusion (defined as more than 10 units within 6 hours), and to die of exsanguination [68]. However, 64% of patients were in fibrinolysis shutdown and were more likely to die of multiorgan failure [68]. Fibrinolysis shutdown is the state in which a patient shows less than the physiologic amount of fibrinolysis (ie, the body's ability to remove unnecessary clots is compromised) and was defined by Moore and colleagues [68] as an LY30 less than 0.8%. The question raised by these results is whether the administration of an antifibrinolytic, such as tranexamic acid, would worsen outcomes in patients who are not in hyperfibrinolysis.

Recent discussion has suggested possible benefits from the early administration of platelets in the setting of expected massive transfusion. There was a reduction in mortality caused by exsanguination in the group that received a higher amount of fresh frozen plasma and platelets in the first 24 hours in the Pragmatic, Randomized Optimal Platelet and Plasma Ratios (PROPPR) study [79]. One of the criticisms of the study is that the group with the survival advantage received platelets earlier, which could be a potential confounder [80].

Therefore, the early administration of platelets may be causing the reduction in exsanguination, not the ratio of platelets and plasma to blood cells. Note that Moore and colleagues [72] have found that lysed platelets, when mixed with whole blood, inhibit the function of tPA similarly to what is seen in fibrinolysis shutdown. If fibrinolysis shutdown occurred because of the administration of platelets, the expected findings would be a reduction in hemorrhage and a possible increase in multiple organ failure. A review from 2013 found insufficient evidence to strongly support the liberal administration of platelets. However, there is a reported mortality benefit for higher ratios of platelet to blood transfusion in the setting of a massive transfusion [81]. The same review also found 2 studies that reported a higher rate of multiple organ failure with the higher ratio of platelet transfusion [81]. The last question left unanswered is the cause of fibrinolysis shutdown, and whether it is platelet mediated.

One promising area of research has been the use of tranexamic acid in traumatic brain injury. Two underpowered prospective studies have already been published [82,83] and an analysis of their combined results showed a trend toward reduced in-hospital mortality and improvement in functional status, as well as a statistically significant reduction in the progression of intracranial hemorrhage [84]. A retrospective study on pediatric patients also observed higher Glasgow Coma Scale scores in patients who had received tranexamic acid [75]. Multiple other prospective studies are currently underway to investigate the benefit of tranexamic acid in traumatic brain injury.

DAMAGE CONTROL RESUSCITATION

Although the techniques for damage control surgery have been described since the 1970s, the first truncated laparotomy in the presence of coagulopathy was described by Stone and colleagues [85] in 1983. This technique was formalized by Rotondo and colleagues [86], who described a tiered approach to caring for patients with exsanguinating injury. Schreiber [55] stated that, "The philosophy of damage control dictates abbreviation of the operations before the development of physiologic exhaustion." Because damage control surgery is a response to the development of exsanguinating hemorrhage and coagulopathy, it is illogical to discuss damage control resuscitation as a discrete entity. It is a focus on the medical contribution of a team model to the care of a patient in extremis in which the anesthesiologist has an important role.

Ideally, patients who could benefit from damage control surgery (ie, rapid control of hemorrhage and contamination) would be identified early. Suggested criteria are listed in Box 2 and may serve as a reference during continued resuscitation to help guide the overall management of individual patients. These patients may characteristically be hypotensive, tachycardic, dyspneic, or in an altered mental state [87]. Rapid correction of acidosis, hypothermia, and coagulopathy during initial resuscitation of the traumatically injured in the setting of hemorrhage control provides the opportunity to avoid a staged damage control procedure [59].

One of the goals of damage control resuscitation is to correct acidosis and improve lactate clearance, because higher levels of serum lactate are associated

Box 2: Factors for considering damage control surgery

Conditions

- High-energy blunt torso trauma
- Multiple torso penetrations
- Hemodynamic instability
- Presenting coagulopathy and/or hypothermia

Complexes

- Major abdominal vascular injury with multiple visceral injuries
- Multifocal or multicavitary exsanguination with concomitant visceral injuries
- Multiregional injury with competing priorities

Critical factors

- Severe metabolic acidosis (pH <7.20)
- Base deficit greater than 15
- Hypothermia (temperature <35°C)
- Resuscitation and operative time more than 90 minutes
- Coagulopathy as shown by development of nonmechanical bleeding
- Massive transfusion (>10 units of packed red blood cells)

Adapted from Refs [59,84,87].

with higher mortality [87–89]. Volume resuscitation should be accompanied by vasodilation with analgesics and/or anesthetics to maintain a systolic blood pressure of 90 mm Hg [88,90], except in the case of traumatic brain injury. This approach allows perfusion of vascular beds that are ischemic from the intense vasoconstriction associated with hemorrhagic shock. There is some thought that the lower blood pressure prevents clot disruption and reduces blood loss [60,88,89]. The recommended packed red blood cell to plasma ratio is between 1:1 and 1:2 [79].

Hypothermia is also associated with increased mortality, and an important goal of damage control resuscitation is the maintenance or return of normothermia [87,88]. In addition, resuscitation should correct clinically significant coagulopathy [86]. Damage control resuscitation focuses on tailoring resuscitation to laboratory findings and limiting crystalloid infusions to the patient [55,59,88]. Multiple different derangements in coagulation may be present (eg, thrombocytopenia, platelet dysfunction, hyperfibrinolysis, hypofibrinogenemia), thus point-of-care viscoelastic tests should be used, because they provide better and more prompt results than standard coagulation panels [64,65]. In the setting of hyperfibrinolysis, an antifibrinolytic should be administered because this has been shown to decrease mortality in trauma. In animal models, fluid resuscitation with plasma instead of crystalloid decreases the incidence of hyperfibrinolysis and decreases mortality [91], which may be why there is evidence for lower mortality with higher frozen fresh plasma to packed red blood cell ratios of transfusions [79,92]. Besides using blood products, factor concentrates can correct coagulation derangements and limit the volume that is administered to the patient [55]. Thus, administration of blood products and coagulants should be based on laboratory findings when available to avoid overcorrection and potential complications associated with their administration [80]. However, in the absence of laboratory findings and in the setting of ongoing hemorrhage suggesting coagulopathy, or in the setting of uncontrolled hemorrhage with the anticipation of a massive transfusion, the early use of plasma and platelets should be encouraged in a balanced ratio with packed red blood cells in the initial resuscitation of patients with trauma.

SUMMARY

Since trauma continues to be a leading cause of morbidity and mortality, it is crucial for anesthesiologists to have experience and expertise in caring for patients with trauma. The airway remains at the top of the list of priorities when treating patients who have significant injuries. Proper airway management with cervical spine immobilization is indicated for any patient who has persistent hypoxemia, severe cognitive impairment, or hypoventilation [10]. However, depending on the experience level of the prehospital provider, airway management does not have to mean intubation. Bag-valve-mask ventilation and placement of supraglottic devices can be very effective techniques for oxygenating and ventilating patients. Apneic oxygenation, in addition to the more common use of preoxygenation, can increase the time available to safely secure the airway, especially in high-risk patients. A rapid thromboelastogram can give a faster and more accurate understanding of overall hemostasis status in patients with trauma than can more traditional coagulation tests. The use of antifibrinolytics in trauma has been supported by various studies, and ongoing research is examining the effect of tranexamic acid in trauma and traumatic brain injury. In the most severely injured patients, the focus is on damage control resuscitation (the correction of acidosis, coagulopathy, shock, and hypothermia) while surgeons perform abbreviated operations targeted to immediately life-threatening injury. Close communication between the surgical and anesthesia teams is necessary for optimum resuscitation and restoration of end-organ integrity.

References

[1] Kauvar DS, Lefering R, Wade CE. Impact of haemorrhage on trauma outcome: an overview of epidemiology, clinical presentations, and therapeutic considerations. J Trauma 2006;60(6 Suppl):S3–11.

[2] Committee on Trauma American College of Surgeons. Collaborative clinical services. In: Rotondo MF, Cribari C, Smith RS, editors. Resources for optimal care of the injured patient. Chicago: American College of Surgeons; 2014. p. 76–87.

[3] Varon AJ, Hagberg CA. The need for a trauma anesthesiology director at level 1 trauma centers. American Society of Anesthesiologists Article 2015;79(6):10–2. Available at: http://monitor.pubs.asahq.org/article.aspx?articleid=2434527. Accessed February 14, 2016.
[4] Brohi K, Cohen MJ, Davenport RA. Acute coagulopathy of trauma: mechanism, identification and effect. Curr Opin Crit Care 2007;13:680–5.
[5] ATLS Subcommittee, American College of Surgeons' Committee on Trauma, International ATLS Working Group. Advanced trauma life support (ATLS®): the ninth edition. J Trauma Acute Care Surg 2013;74:1363–6.
[6] Garcia A. Critical care issues in the early management of severe trauma. Surg Clin North Am 2006;86:1359–87.
[7] Gruen RL, Jurkovich GJ, McIntyre LK, et al. Patterns of errors contributing to trauma mortality: lessons learned from 2,594 deaths. Ann Surg 2006;244:371–80.
[8] Miraflor E, Chuang K, Miranda MA, et al. Timing is everything: delayed intubation is associated with increased mortality in initially stable trauma patients. J Surg Res 2011;170:286–90.
[9] Teixeira PG, Inaba K, Hadjizacharia P, et al. Preventable or potentially preventable mortality at a mature trauma center. J Trauma 2007;63:1338–46 [discussion: 46–7].
[10] Mayglothling J, Duane TM, Gibbs M, et al. Emergency tracheal intubation immediately following traumatic injury: an Eastern Association for the Surgery of Trauma practice management guideline. J Trauma Acute Care Surg 2012;73:S333–40.
[11] Apfelbaum JL, Hagberg CA, Caplan RA, et al. Practice guidelines for management of the difficult airway: an updated report by the American Society of Anesthesiologists Task Force on Management of the Difficult Airway. Anesthesiology 2013;118:251–70.
[12] Stephens CT, Kahntroff S, Dutton RP. The success of emergency endotracheal intubation in trauma patients: a 10-year experience at a major adult trauma referral center. Anesth Analg 2009;109:866–72.
[13] Horton CL, Brown CA 3rd, Raja AS. Trauma airway management. J Emerg Med 2014;46:814–20.
[14] Martini RP, Larson DM. Clinical evaluation and airway management for adults with cervical spine instability. Anesthesiol Clin 2015;33:315–27.
[15] Santoni BG, Hindman BJ, Puttlitz CM, et al. Manual in-line stabilization increases pressures applied by the laryngoscope blade during direct laryngoscopy and orotracheal intubation. Anesthesiology 2009;110:24–31.
[16] Bathory I, Frascarolo P, Kern C, et al. Evaluation of the GlideScope for tracheal intubation in patients with cervical spine immobilisation by a semi-rigid collar. Anaesthesia 2009;64:1337–41.
[17] Sakles JC, Mosier JM, Chiu S, et al. Tracheal intubation in the emergency department: a comparison of GlideScope® video laryngoscopy to direct laryngoscopy in 822 intubations. J Emerg Med 2012;42:400–5.
[18] Malik MA, Maharaj CH, Harte BH, et al. Comparison of Macintosh, Truview EVO2, Glidescope, and Airwayscope laryngoscope use in patients with cervical spine immobilization. Br J Anaesth 2008;101:723–30.
[19] Maruyama K, Yamada T, Kawakami R, et al. Randomized cross-over comparison of cervical-spine motion with the AirWay Scope or Macintosh laryngoscope with in-line stabilization: a video-fluoroscopic study. Br J Anaesth 2008;101:563–7.
[20] Kill C, Risse J, Wallot P, et al. Videolaryngoscopy with Glidescope reduces cervical spine movement in patients with unsecured cervical spine. J Emerg Med 2013;44:750–6.
[21] Gavrilovska-Brzanov A, Jarallah MA, Cogliati A, et al. Evaluation of the hemodynamic response to endotracheal intubation comparing the Airtraq® with Macintosh laryngoscopes in cardiac surgical patients. Acta Inform Med 2015;23:280–4.
[22] Tempe DK, Chaudhary K, Diwakar A, et al. Comparison of hemodynamic responses to laryngoscopy and intubation with Truview PCD™, McGrath® and Macintosh laryngoscope

in patients undergoing coronary artery bypass grafting: a randomized prospective study. Ann Card Anaesth 2016;19:68–75.
[23] Wetsch WA, Spelten O, Hellmich M, et al. Comparison of different video laryngoscopes for emergency intubation in a standardized airway manikin with immobilized cervical spine by experienced anaesthetists. A randomized, controlled crossover trial. Resuscitation 2012;83:740–5.
[24] Kaplan A, Göksu E, Yıldız G, et al. Comparison of the C-MAC video laryngoscope and rigid fiberscope with direct laryngoscopy in easy and difficult airway scenarios: a manikin study. J Emerg Med 2016;50:e107–14.
[25] Ruetzler K, Imach S, Weiss M, et al. Comparison of five video laryngoscopes and conventional direct laryngoscopy: investigations on simple and simulated difficult airways on the intubation trainer. Anaesthesist 2015;64:513–9 [in German].
[26] Sun DA, Warriner CB, Parsons DG, et al. The GlideScope Video Laryngoscope: randomized clinical trial in 200 patients. Br J Anaesth 2005;94:381–4.
[27] Jain U, McCunn M, Smith CE, et al. Management of the traumatized airway. Anesthesiology 2016;124:199–206.
[28] Bernard SA, Nguyen V, Cameron P, et al. Prehospital rapid sequence intubation improves functional outcome for patients with severe traumatic brain injury: a randomized controlled trial. Ann Surg 2010;252:959–65.
[29] Bukur M, Kurtovic S, Berry C, et al. Pre-hospital intubation is associated with increased mortality after traumatic brain injury. J Surg Res 2011;170:e117–21.
[30] Stockinger ZT, McSwain NE Jr. Prehospital endotracheal intubation for trauma does not improve survival over bag-valve-mask ventilation. J Trauma 2004;56:531–6.
[31] Seamon MJ, Fisher CA, Gaughan J, et al. Prehospital procedures before emergency department thoracotomy: "scoop and run" saves lives. J Trauma 2007;63:113–20.
[32] Cobas MA, De la Peña MA, Manning R, et al. Prehospital intubations and mortality: a level 1 trauma center perspective. Anesth Analg 2009;109:489–93.
[33] Tentillier E, Heydenreich C, Cros AM, et al. Use of the intubating laryngeal mask airway in emergency pre-hospital difficult intubation. Resuscitation 2008;77:30–4.
[34] Davis DP, Koprowicz KM, Newgard CD, et al. The relationship between out-of-hospital airway management and outcome among trauma patients with Glasgow Coma Scale scores of 8 or less. Prehosp Emerg Care 2011;15:184–92.
[35] Lossius HM, Roislien J, Lockey DJ. Patient safety in pre-hospital emergency tracheal intubation: a comprehensive meta-analysis of the intubation success rates of EMS providers. Crit Care 2012;16:R24.
[36] Breckwoldt J, Klemstein S, Brunne B, et al. Expertise in prehospital endotracheal intubation by emergency medicine physicians–Comparing 'proficient performers' and 'experts'. Resuscitation 2012;83:434–9.
[37] Taghavi S, Jayarajan SN, Khoche S, et al. Examining prehospital intubation for penetrating trauma in a swine hemorrhagic shock model. J Trauma Acute Care Surg 2013;74:1246–51.
[38] von Goedecke A, Herff H, Paal P, et al. Field airway management disasters. Anesth Analg 2007;104:481–3.
[39] Herff H, Wenzel V, Lockey D. Prehospital intubation: the right tools in the right hands at the right time. Anesth Analg 2009;109:303–5.
[40] Kempema J, Trust MD, Ali S, et al. Prehospital endotracheal intubation vs extraglottic airway device in blunt trauma. Am J Emerg Med 2015;33:1080–3.
[41] Bosch J, de Nooij J, de Visser M, et al. Prehospital use in emergency patients of a laryngeal mask airway by ambulance paramedics is a safe and effective alternative for endotracheal intubation. Emerg Med J 2014;31:750–3.
[42] Lecky F, Bryden D, Little R, et al. Emergency intubation for acutely ill and injured patients. Cochrane Database Syst Rev 2008;(2):CD001429.

[43] Lockey DJ, Crewdson K, Lossius HM. Pre-hospital anaesthesia: the same but different. Br J Anaesth 2014;113:211–9.
[44] Frumin MJ, Epstein RM, Cohen G. Apneic oxygenation in man. Anesthesiology 1959;20: 20789–98.
[45] Ramachandran SK, Cosnowski A, Shanks A, et al. Apneic oxygenation during prolonged laryngoscopy in obese patients: a randomized, controlled trial of nasal oxygen administration. J Clin Anesth 2010;22:164–8.
[46] Semler MW, Janz DR, Lentz RJ, et al. Randomized trial of apneic oxygenation during endotracheal intubation of the critically ill. Am J Respir Crit Care Med 2016;193:273–80.
[47] Miguel-Montanes R, Hajage D, Messika J, et al. Use of high-flow nasal cannula oxygen therapy to prevent desaturation during tracheal intubation of intensive care patients with mild-to-moderate hypoxemia. Crit Care Med 2015;43:574–83.
[48] Teller LE, Alexander CM, Frumin MJ, et al. Pharyngeal insufflation of oxygen prevents arterial desaturation during apnea. Anesthesiology 1988;69:980–2.
[49] Frerk C, Mitchell VS, McNarry AF, et al. Difficult Airway Society 2015 guidelines for management of unanticipated difficult intubation in adults. Br J Anaesth 2015;115:827–48.
[50] Sauaia A, Moore FA, Moore EE, et al. Epidemiology of trauma deaths: a reassessment. J Trauma 1995;38:185–93.
[51] Maegele M, Lefering R, Yucel N, et al. Early coagulopathy in multiple injury: an analysis from the German Trauma Registry on 8724 patients. Injury 2007;38:298–304.
[52] Kutcher ME, Ferguson AR, Cohen MJ. A principal component analysis of coagulation after trauma. J Trauma Acute Care Surg 2013;74:1223–9 [discussion: 1229–30].
[53] Brohi K, Singh J, Heron M, et al. Acute traumatic coagulopathy. J Trauma 2003;54(6): 1127–30.
[54] Schreiber MA. Damage control surgery. Crit Care Clin 2004;20:101–18.
[55] Schreiber MA. The beginning of the end for damage control surgery. Br J Surg 2012;99(Suppl 1):10–1.
[56] DeLoughery TG. Coagulation defects in trauma patients: etiology, recognition, and therapy. Crit Care Clin 2004;20:13–24.
[57] Brohi K, Cohen MJ, Ganter MT, et al. Acute coagulopathy of trauma: hypoperfusion induces systemic anticoagulation and hyperfibrinolysis. J Trauma 2008;64:1211–7.
[58] Frith D, Goslings JC, Gaarder C, et al. Definition and drivers of acute traumatic coagulopathy: clinical and experimental investigations. J Thromb Haemost 2010;8:1919–25.
[59] Ball CG. Damage control resuscitation: history, theory and technique [review]. Can J Surg 2014;57:55–60.
[60] Pawelczyk NS, Huby Mdel P, Salsbury JR, et al. Association of hemodilution and blood pressure in uncontrolled bleeding. J Surg Res 2013;184:959–65.
[61] Segal JB, Dzik WH, Transfusion Medicine/Hemostasis Clinical Trials Network. Paucity of studies to support that abnormal coagulation test results predict bleeding in the setting of invasive procedures: an evidence-based review. Transfusion 2005;45:1413–25.
[62] Kitchens CS. To bleed or not to bleed? Is that the question for the PTT? J Thromb Haemost 2005;3:2607–11.
[63] Haas T, Fries D, Tanaka KA, et al. Usefulness of standard plasma coagulation tests in the management of perioperative coagulopathic bleeding: is there any evidence? Br J Anaesth 2015;114:217–24.
[64] Holcomb JB, Minei KM, Scerbo ML, et al. Admission rapid thrombelastography can replace conventional coagulation tests in the emergency department: experience with 1974 consecutive trauma patients. Ann Surg 2012;256:476–86.
[65] Plotkin AJ, Wade CE, Jenkins DH, et al. A reduction in clot formation rate and strength assessed by thrombelastography is indicative of transfusion requirements in patients with penetrating injuries. J Trauma 2008;64:S64–8.

[66] Cotton BA, Harvin JA, Kostousouv V, et al. Hyperfibrinolysis at admission is an uncommon but highly lethal event associated with shock and prehospital fluid administration. J Trauma Acute Care Surg 2012;73:365–70 [discussion: 370].
[67] Chapman MP, Moore EE, Ramos CR, et al. Fibrinolysis greater than 3% is the critical value for initiation of antifibrinolytic therapy. J Trauma Acute Care Surg 2013;75:961–7 [discussion: 967].
[68] Moore HB, Moore EE, Gonzalez E, et al. Hyperfibrinolysis, physiologic fibrinolysis, and fibrinolysis shutdown: the spectrum of postinjury fibrinolysis and relevance to antifibrinolytic therapy. J Trauma Acute Care Surg 2014;77:811–7 [discussion: 817].
[69] Jeger V, Willi S, Liu T, et al. The Rapid TEG α-Angle may be a sensitive predictor of transfusion in moderately injured blunt trauma patients. ScientificWorldJournal 2012;2012: 821794.
[70] Lee TH, McCully BH, Underwood SJ, et al. Correlation of conventional thrombelastography and rapid thrombelastography in trauma. Am J Surg 2013;205:521–7 [discussion: 527].
[71] Moore HB, Moore EE, Chapman MP, et al. Viscoelastic measurements of platelet function, not fibrinogen function, predicts sensitivity to tissue-type plasminogen activator in trauma patients. J Thromb Haemost 2015;13:1878–87.
[72] Moore HB, Moore EE, Gonzalez E, et al. Hemolysis exacerbates hyperfibrinolysis, whereas platelolysis shuts down fibrinolysis: evolving concepts of the spectrum of fibrinolysis in response to severe injury. Shock 2015;43:39–46.
[73] Shakur H, Roberts I, Bautista R, et al. Effects of tranexamic acid on death, vascular occlusive events, and blood transfusion in trauma patients with significant haemorrhage (CRASH-2): a randomised, placebo-controlled trial. Lancet 2010;376:23–32.
[74] Cole E, Davenport R, Willett K, et al. Tranexamic acid use in severely injured civilian patients and the effects on outcomes: a prospective cohort study. Ann Surg 2015;261:390–4.
[75] Eckert MJ, Wertin TM, Tyner SD, et al. Tranexamic acid administration to pediatric trauma patients in a combat setting: the pediatric trauma and tranexamic acid study (PED-TRAX). J Trauma Acute Care Surg 2014;77:852–8 [discussion: 858].
[76] Perel P, Ker K, Morales Uribe CH, et al. Tranexamic acid for reducing mortality in emergency and urgent surgery. Cochrane Database Syst Rev 2013;(1):CD010245.
[77] Napolitano LM, Cohen MJ, Cotton BA, et al. Tranexamic acid in trauma: how should we use it? J Trauma Acute Care Surg 2013;74:1575–86.
[78] Raza I, Davenport R, Rourke C, et al. The incidence and magnitude of fibrinolytic activation in trauma patients. J Thromb Haemost 2013;11:307–14.
[79] Holcomb JB, Tilley BC, Baraniuk S, et al. Transfusion of plasma, platelets, and red blood cells in a 1:1:1 vs a 1:1:2 ratio and mortality in patients with severe trauma: the PROPPR randomized clinical trial. JAMA 2015;313:471–82.
[80] Janelle GM, Shore-Lesserson L, Smith CE, et al. What is the PROPPR transfusion strategy in trauma resuscitation? Anesth Analg 2016;122(4):1216–9.
[81] Hallet J, Lauzier F, Mailloux O, et al. The use of higher platelet: RBC transfusion ratio in the acute phase of trauma resuscitation: a systematic review. Crit Care Med 2013;41(12): 2800–11.
[82] CRASH-2 Collaborators, Intracranial Bleeding Study. Effect of tranexamic acid in traumatic brain injury: a nested randomised, placebo controlled trial (CRASH-2 Intracranial Bleeding Study). BMJ 2011;343:d3795.
[83] Yutthakasemsunt S, Kittiwatanagul W, Piyavechvirat P, et al. Tranexamic acid for patients with traumatic brain injury: a randomized, double-blinded, placebo-controlled trial. BMC Emerg Med 2013;13:20.
[84] Zehtabchi S, Abdel Baki SG, Falzon L, et al. Tranexamic acid for traumatic brain injury: a systematic review and meta-analysis. Am J Emerg Med 2014;32:1503–9.
[85] Stone HH, Strom PR, Mullins RJ. Management of the major coagulopathy with onset during laparotomy. Ann Surg 1983;197:532–5.

[86] Rotondo MF, Schwab CW, McGonigal MD, et al. 'Damage control': an approach for improved survival in exsanguinating penetrating abdominal injury. J Trauma 1993;35: 375–82 [discussion: 382–3].
[87] Rotondo MF, Zonies DH. The damage control sequence and underlying logic. Surg Clin North Am 1997;77:761–77.
[88] Holcomb JB. Damage control resuscitation. J Trauma 2007;62:S36–7.
[89] Connelly CR, Schreiber MA. Endpoints in resuscitation. Curr Opin Crit Care 2015;21: 512–9.
[90] Dutton RP. Anesthesia during resuscitation: panacea or poison? Trauma Anesthesiology Society; 2016. Available at: https://tas.ucsf.edu/doc/2016-01_Dutton.pdf. Accessed March 17, 2016.
[91] Moore HB, Moore EE, Morton AP, et al. Shock-induced systemic hyperfibrinolysis is attenuated by plasma-first resuscitation. J Trauma Acute Care Surg 2015;79:897–903.
[92] del Junco DJ, Holcomb JB, Fox EE, et al. Resuscitate early with plasma and platelets or balance blood products gradually: findings from the PROMMTT study. J Trauma Acute Care Surg 2013;75(1 Suppl 1):S24–30.

Advances in Anesthesia 34 (2016) 29–46

ADVANCES IN ANESTHESIA

New Developments in Cardiac Arrest Management

Matthias L. Riess, MD, PhD[a,b,c,*]

[a]Department of Anesthesiology, Vanderbilt University, 1161 21st Avenue South, T4202 MCN, Nashville, TN 37232-2520, USA; [b]Department of Pharmacology, Vanderbilt University, 2220 Pierce Avenue, Nashville, TN 37232, USA; [c]Department of Anesthesiology, TVHS VA Medical Center, 1310 24th Avenue South, Nashville, TN 37212, USA

Keywords

• ACLS guidelines • Active compression/decompression
• Cardiopulmonary resuscitation • Impedance threshold device • Postconditioning

Key points

- Cardiac arrest continues to be a substantial health care problem worldwide because of its combination of high frequency and low rate of neurologically favorable survival.
- Immediate and high-quality cardiopulmonary resuscitation remains the focus of the most current 2015 ACLS guidelines and of substantial system-based, educational, clinical, and translational research efforts.
- Mechanical adjunct devices, such as active compression/decompression or automated chest compression devices, in combination with an impedance threshold device aim to improve cerebral blood flow and survival.
- High-quality CPR is absolutely necessary to benefit the patient when using an impedance threshold device.
- Perioperative cardiac arrest is rare and its management is largely etiology-driven.
- Endtidal carbon dioxide measurement helps improve resuscitative efforts, recognize return of spontaneous circulation, and can add to prognostication.
- Postarrest targeted temperature management and postconditioning strategies aim to ameliorate cerebral ischemia-reperfusion injury.

Disclosure Statement: The author has no conflict of interest. He receives research funding from the National Institutes of Health (5R01 HL123227).

*Department of Anesthesiology, 1161 21st Avenue South, T4202 MCN, Nashville, TN 37232-2520. *E-mail address:* matthias.riess@vanderbilt.edu

http://dx.doi.org/10.1016/j.aan.2016.07.003
0737-6146/16/Published by Elsevier Inc.

INTRODUCTION

Cardiac arrest continues to be a substantial health care problem worldwide because of its combination of high frequency and low survival. In the United States alone, an estimated 350,000 out-of-hospital cardiac arrests (OHCA) occur every year [1], with similarly high numbers in Europe [2]. Despite significant regional variations, overall chances for functionally favorable survival remain low, between 5% and 10% [3,4]. According to the Cardiac Arrest Registry to Enhance Survival, patients with OHCA are on average 64 ± 18 years old, 61% are male, and 22% are pronounced dead before arrival at the hospital [5]. Only about one-third receive cardiopulmonary resuscitation (CPR) by bystanders, and less than 4% are treated with an automated external defibrillator before the arrival of emergency medical service personnel. A cardiac cause has been described in 70% to 85% of OHCA; the remainder is a consequence of noncardiac causes, such as trauma, drowning, overdose, asphyxia, electrocution, primary respiratory arrests, or other etiologies. The highest survival rates are achieved when the arrest is witnessed by a bystander and the patient has a shockable rhythm, such as pulseless ventricular tachycardia or ventricular fibrillation (VF). Thus, predictors of OHCA survival (Table 1) are (1) witnessed by a bystander, (2) witnessed by emergency medical service, (3) bystander CPR, (4) shockable cardiac rhythm (only 23% of all OHCAs), and (5) return of spontaneous circulation (ROSC) in the field [6].

The situation for in-hospital cardiac arrest (IHCA) differs only marginally. According to the British registry [7], the incidence of IHCA is estimated to be 1.6 per 1000 hospital admissions, with 17% being in a shockable rhythm versus 72% in asystole or pulseless electrical activity. Overall survival rates have improved from 10% in the 1950s to 17% in the 1990s. A large-scale study, however, has reported a plateau of the overall average survival-to-discharge rate at 18% [8], comprising 49% for shockable rhythms, but only 11% for nonshockable rhythms. About half of the IHCA occur on regular wards, between 5% and 10% in intensive care and coronary care units. Predictors for survival of IHCA (Table 2) are (1) witnessed arrest, (2) initial rhythm shockable, (3) epinephrine dose administered within 2 minutes of arrest, and (4) arrest in the intensive care unit rather than on the ward [9].

Table 1
Predictors of survival after out-of-hospital cardiac arrest

Predictors of survival	Survival probability, %
Witnessed by a bystander	6.4–13.5
Bystander CPR	3.9–16.1
Witnessed by EMS personnel	4.9–18.2
Initial rhythm shockable	14.8–23.0
Return of spontaneous circulation in the field	15.5–33.6

Abbreviation: EMS, emergency medical system.

Adapted from Sasson C, Rogers MA, Dahl J, et al. Predictors of survival from out-of-hospital cardiac arrest: a systematic review and meta-analysis. Circ Cardiovasc Qual Outcomes 2010;3(1):63–81.

Table 2
Predictors of survival after in-hospital cardiac arrest

Predictors of survival	Survival probability, %
Initial rhythm shockable	85
Arrest in the intensive care unit	56
Epinephrine administered within 2 min of arrest	54
Witnessed arrest	52

Adapted from Fennelly NK, McPhillips C, Gilligan P. Arrest in hospital: a study of in hospital cardiac arrest outcomes. Ir Med J 2014;107(4):105–7.

Perioperative cardiac arrests are rare. Their incidence is estimated to be about 7.4 per 10,000 anesthetics with the risk of death from cardiac arrest attributable to anesthesia being 0.6 per 10,000 anesthetics [10]. Risk factors for perioperative cardiac arrest include older age; male gender; American Society of Anesthesiologists physical status of IV or higher; upper abdominal, thoracic, spine, and/or emergency surgery; longer and after hours procedures; and general versus nongeneral anesthesia [10]. Although the cause of OHCA and even IHCA is often unknown the list of probable causes for cardiac arrest in the perioperative period is more succinct (Box 1) [11].

Overall, the public health burden of cardiac arrest remains immense. A reasonable analogy of the impact of cardiac arrest on public health are two full Boeing 747 aircraft crashing with total loss of life per day on each continent [2]. With recent discoveries and insights into improved resuscitation technique, overall functionally favorable survival rate could be improved and a proportion of this premature death prevented. This article highlights some important recent developments in the area of cardiocerebral resuscitation after cardiac arrest.

HISTORY OF CARDIOPULMONARY RESUSCITATION

In 1958, Safar [12] described effective pulmonary ventilation by mouth-to-mouth breathing without an artificial airway. In 1960, Kouwenhoven and coworkers [13] for the first time documented 14 cardiac arrest victims who were successfully treated with closed chest cardiac massage and survived. In the same year, the Maryland Medical Society introduced the combination of chest compressions and rescue breathing, the foundation of what is recognized today as CPR [14]. In 1962, Lown and colleagues [15] described for the first time direct-current, monophasic waveform defibrillation. Four years later, the American Heart Association (AHA) developed the first CPR guidelines, which since then have been updated regularly. The process of generating CPR guidelines has evolved over several decades. The AHA, the European Resuscitation Council, the Heart and Stroke Foundation of Canada, the Australian Resuscitation Council, and others have been comprehensively evaluating the available resuscitation science and collaborating extensively for decades, which has led to similar CPR guidelines published in different regions of the world.

Box 1: Common causes of perioperative cardiac arrest

Cardiovascular

High parasympathetic tone: vagal reflex, electroconvulsive therapy

Hypovolemia/hemorrhage

Embolism: thrombi, gas, cement

Increased intra-abdominal pressure

Anaphylaxis/transfusion reaction

Pulmonary hypertension

Acute coronary syndrome

Pacemaker failure

Electrolyte imbalance: hyperkalemia, hypocalcemia

Respiratory

Hypoxemia/hypercarbia

Increased intrathoracic pressure: bronchospasm, auto positive end-expiratory pressure, tension pneumothorax

Anesthesia

Anesthetic overdose

High neuroaxial block with sympathectomy

Local anesthetic toxicity

Malignant hyperthermia

Drug errors

Adapted from Moitra VK, Gabrielli A, Maccioli GA, et al. Anesthesia advanced circulatory life support. Can J Anaesth 2012;59(6):586–603.

The most current (2015) AHA Advanced Cardiac Life Support (ACLS) guidelines (www.heart.org/eccguidelines) stress several key points (Box 2, Fig. 1) [16]: (1) early defibrillation and early chest compressions; (2) high-quality compressions, that is, a rate of 100–120 compressions per minute, a compression depth of at least 2 inches, and complete chest recoil; (3) no unnecessary interruptions of chest compressions; and (4) a ventilation rate no greater than 8 to 10 breaths per minute. The scientific basis for these recommendations is outlined next.

EARLY CHEST COMPRESSIONS AND EARLY DEFIBRILLATION

To achieve ROSC, early CPR and defibrillation are critical for survival when a shockable rhythm is encountered. Defibrillation is the best treatment of VF cardiac arrest because with immediate CPR survival rates decrease by only 3% to 4% per minute, whereas without immediate CPR this rate is 7% to 10% per minute.

Box 2: Important features of current (2015) CPR guidelines

High-quality chest compressions

- Compression rate at 100 to 120[a] per minute
- Compression depth at least 2 inches
- Complete recoil

Uninterrupted chest compressions

- Start with compressions
- Only one shock at a time followed by immediate CPR

Avoid excessive ventilation

- 30:2 compression/ventilation ratio for single rescuers of adults, children, and infants
- Advanced airway: continuous chest compressions, ventilation every 6 to 8 seconds

Removal of vasopressin from algorithm[a]

[a] Different from 2010 guidelines.

Adapted from Link MS, Berkow LC, Kudenchuk PJ, et al. Part 7: adult advanced cardiovascular life support: 2015 American Heart Association guidelines update for cardiopulmonary resuscitation and emergency cardiovascular care. Circulation 2015;132(18 Suppl 2):S444–64.

Therefore, CPR can double to triple survival, not only by providing blood flow to vital organs, but also by prolonging VF and delaying the onset of asystole, thus extending the window for successful defibrillation [17].

HIGH-QUALITY CHEST COMPRESSIONS

The highest rates of ROSC and survival are achieved at chest compression rates between 100 and 120 per minute [18]. Compression depth is linearly related to survival, with chest compressions of only 1 inch depth instead of 2 inches resulting in 50% lower survival rates as reported by Edelson and colleagues [19]. Compression depths of more than 2.4 inches, however, should be avoided because of increased risk for injury [20]. Equally important as sufficient compression depth is complete recoil to a neutral sternum position on the upstroke of CPR. Incomplete chest recoil leads to increased intrathoracic pressure, which in turn increases intracerebral pressure and decreases filling of the right heart with subsequently lower cardiac output, both of which synergistically reduce cerebral blood flow [21,22]. Incomplete recoil or "leaning" is prevented with appropriate training [23] and an optimal hand technique [22].

PRIORITIZING CHEST COMPRESSIONS AND MINIMIZING PAUSES

Blood flow is now prioritized over ventilation. The study by Edelson and colleagues [19] suggests that chest compressions should not be interrupted for

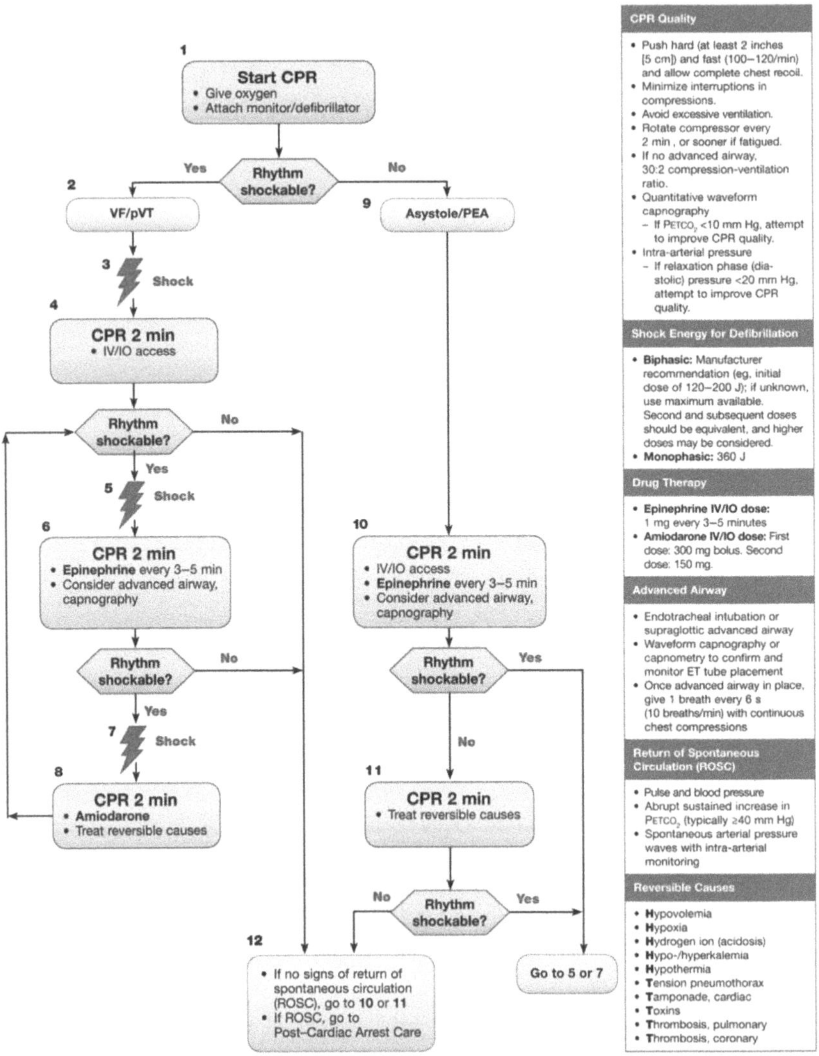

Fig. 1. 2015 CPR guidelines according to the American Heart Association. ET, endotracheal tube; IO, intraosseous; IV, intravenous; PEA, pulseless electrical activity; pVT, pulseless ventricular tachycardia. (*From* Link MS, Berkow LC, Kudenchuk PJ, et al. Part 7: adult advanced cardiovascular life support: 2015 American Heart Association guidelines update for cardiopulmonary resuscitation and emergency cardiovascular care. Circulation 2015;132(18 Suppl 2):S452; with permission.)

more than 10 seconds; preshock pauses of 30 seconds, for example, led to a 60% lower success of a subsequent shock compared with pauses less than 10 seconds. This resulted in a fundamental guideline change from A-B-C to C-A-B: instead of starting with airway assessment (A) and breathing (B), the provider should initiate chest compressions (C) immediately. Biphasic shocks should be delivered only once at a time instead of as previously recommended as a stack of three [16]. When shocks were limited to one time, allowing for immediate continuation of chest compressions instead of prolonged pauses, Rea and colleagues [24] reported a 24% increase in ROSC at hospital arrival and a 40% increase in hospital discharge and 1-year survival. The rationale is that the diminishing probability of a second or third shock to be successful, after the first shock has failed, no longer justifies prolonged pauses.

AVOID HYPERVENTILATION

Just as incomplete recoil should be avoided to not lead to continuously increased intrathoracic pressure, excessive positive pressure ventilation can contribute significantly to a decrease in return of blood to the right heart and to increased intracerebral pressure. Aufderheide and colleagues [25] could show in their landmark porcine study increased intrathoracic pressure over time, rather than the hypocapnia associated with hyperventilation, is responsible for a dramatically reduced survival after cardiac arrest and CPR with hyperventilation. Thus, hyperventilation should be avoided by limiting ventilations to 8 to 10 breaths per minute; metronomes may be considered to guide normoventilation.

ROLE OF ENDTIDAL CARBON DIOXIDE PARTIAL PRESSURE IN RESUSCITATION

Endtidal (ET)CO_2 is the partial pressure of exhaled CO_2 at the end of expiration and determined by CO_2 production, pulmonary blood flow, and alveolar ventilation [16]. Waveform capnography visualizes the actual CO_2 waveform during inspiration and expiration. In contrast to stable cardiovascular conditions where ETCO_2 partial pressure serves to differentiate between hypoventilation, normoventilation, and hyperventilation, the primary determinant of ETCO_2 during and after CPR is pulmonary blood flow, and its value becomes more an indicator of passive cardiac output during chest compressions or active cardiac output after ROSC. Consequently, the ACLS guidelines emphasize the need to improve the quality of chest compressions for ETCO_2 values less than 10 mm Hg (see Fig. 1) [16]; conversely, a sustained increase to greater than 40 mm Hg, especially when abrupt, may be an indicator of ROSC. In intubated and normoventilated patients, failure to achieve more than 10 mm Hg ETCO_2 after 20 minutes CPR might be taken into consideration as one element of a multimodal approach in the decision process when to stop resuscitative efforts; ETCO_2, however, should never be used alone or in nonintubated patients [16].

ADJUNCT DEVICES

Even with the best technique, external chest compressions can only produce about 20% to 30% of the normal cardiac output [26,27]. Limited endurance of the rescuer [28] and the difficulty of providing high-performance CPR during patient transport [29] contributes to decreasing quality of manual chest compressions over time. Two newer adjunct devices work synergistically by more efficiently using the heart and chest to pump blood during CPR through lowering intrathoracic and intracranial pressure to improve cardiac and cerebral blood flow during chest compressions.

ACTIVE COMPRESSION-DECOMPRESSION

A case report of a son rescuing his father after cardiac arrest by using a toilet plunger [30] inspired Lurie [31] to the development of active compression-decompression (ACD), where a suction cup is used to actively decompress the chest after a preceding compression, thus lowering intrathoracic pressure faster, and improving cardiac output and generated systolic pressure when used alone [32]. It is marketed as ResQPUMP (ZOLL Medical Corporation, Chelmsford, MA) in different countries, and recently received Food and Drug Administration approval in the United States.

AUTOMATED CHEST COMPRESSION

Automated chest compressors (Fig. 2) are programmed to not exceed normal sternum levels during decompression. The Lund University Cardiopulmonary Assist System (LUCAS-2; PhysioControl, Redmond, WA) is a newer version of the original LUCAS, is battery-powered, and runs with a constant compression rate of 100 min^{-1}, a force of 600 N, a compression depth of 2 inches, and 1:1 duty cycle [33]. In comparison, AutoPulse (ZOLL Medical Corporation) is a battery-powered compression device that uses a circumferential band to squeeze the entire chest as developed by Halperin and colleagues [34,35]. AutoPulse delivers 80 compressions per minute with an even distribution of the compression across the entire chest, while the compression depth can be

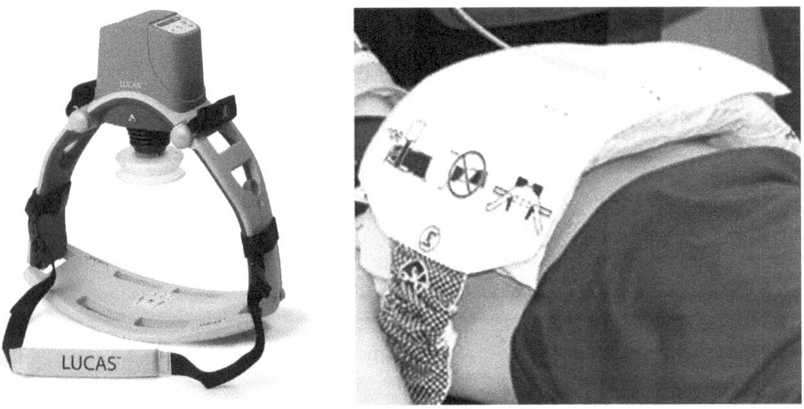

Fig. 2. Examples of automated chest compression devices. LUCAS-2 (*left*); AutoPulse (*right*). (*Courtesy of* [*Left*] Lund University Cardiopulmonary Assist System; PhysioControl, Redmond, WA, with permission; and [*Right*] ZOLL Medical Corporation, Chelmsford, MA; with permission.)

adjusted to the individual patient's chest diameter. For an overview of more mechanical devices from different manufacturers, please refer to recent review articles in this area [33,36]. Earlier studies have reported a higher incidence of rib and sternal fractures after manual ACD versus conventional manual CPR [37]; other case reports have described rare complications, such as tension pneumothorax [38] and liver [39] or splenic lacerations [40]. Nevertheless, neither of these are thought unique to automated versus conventional manual chest compressions [41]. There seem to be, however, subtle differences among devices; Koster and colleagues [42] reported that circumferential compression devices had a higher incidence of visceral damage than LUCAS when compared with manual CPR controls. Clear advantages of mechanical CPR devices are reliable compressions of constant rate, depth, and location, thus avoiding inconsistencies of manual compressions, provider fatigue [43], and injury [44]; at the same time, personnel is freed up for other important tasks (Box 3) [45].

IMPEDANCE THRESHOLD DEVICE

Most importantly, however, the concept of ACD works best in tandem with an impedance threshold device (ITD; Fig. 3; commercially available as ResQPOD, ZOLL Medical Corporation) [46] and vice versa. The ITD creates a small negative intrathoracic pressure during passive chest recoil or active decompression to increase venous return to the heart. The ITD is placed between a tight-sitting face mask or the endotracheal tube on one end, and the ventilation bag or ventilator on the other end as early as possible during CPR. The ITD opens for spontaneous or for positive pressure ventilation and for negative intrathoracic pressures of minus 10 mm Hg or lower. Enhancing venous return to the right heart, ACD and ITD synergistically result in largely improved systemic blood pressures, decreased intracranial pressure, and improved cerebral perfusion during CPR in animal models [46] and in patients [47]. Their combination has been shown to improve neurologically favorable survival in patients with cardiac arrest by 50% on hospital

Box 3: Advantages of mechanical CPR devices

Mechanical CPR devices enable reliable compressions with
- Constant rate
- Constant depth
- Constant location

Mechanical CPR devices avoid
- Inconsistencies of manual compressions
- Provider fatigue
- Injury

Mechanical CPR devices free up personnel for other important tasks

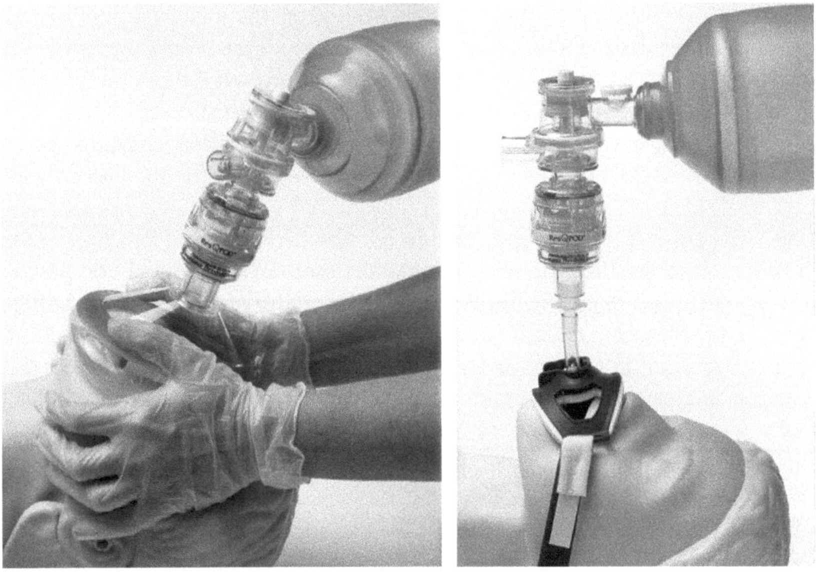

Fig. 3. The impedance threshold device is placed between a tight sitting face mask (*left*) or endotracheal tube (*right*) and the ventilation bag. (*Courtesy of* ZOLL Medical Corporation, Chelmsford, MA; with permission.)

discharge with modified Rankin Scale scores comparable with the control group 1 year later [48].

When used in conjunction with conventional manual CPR alone [49–51], the generation of negative intrathoracic pressure in the presence of an ITD largely depends on the intrinsic elastic recoil of the chest and the quality of CPR. Fractured ribs, for example, or a rigid, noncompliant chest reduce elastic recoil. Moreover, limited recoil through leaning has detrimental physiologic effects on venous return and intracranial pressure as described previously [21,22]. Although the Resuscitation Outcomes Consortium trial with 8718 patients randomly assigned to conventional manual CPR with a sham or an active ITD could not show a benefit of the ITD alone across all-comers [51], a recent post hoc analysis of the data showed a clear benefit in those patients treated with high-quality CPR with regards to a compression rate and depth recommended by the guidelines as opposed to those who did receive CPR outside of the current recommendations [52].

Whether a continuous negative intrathoracic pressure through an intrathoracic pressure regulator by combining an ITD with a vacuum suction to maintain a constant intrathoracic vacuum between minus 5 and 10 mm Hg except during intermittent positive pressure ventilations is an improvement over the ITD during CPR, remains the subject of ongoing animal studies [53–55]. First promising results in humans, however, have been reported during coronary bypass graft surgery [56] and hemorrhagic shock [57].

IMPORTANT CHANGES FROM 2010 AMERICAN HEART ASSOCIATION GUIDELINES

The 2015 AHA guidelines serve less as a comprehensive revision than an update of the 2010 AHA guidelines for CPR and have to be interpreted in this context [58]. Moreover, as of 2015, the guidelines have now moved from periodic revisions and updates every 5 years to a continuously updated World Wide Web–based format (https://eccguidelines.heart.org/) enabling a more rapid translation of new scientific discoveries into daily patient care. Systems of care and continuous quality improvement are important new components that emphasize integrated structures and processes essential for OHCA and IHCA resuscitation capable of measuring quality and improving patient outcomes [59]. Another new feature is education of lay rescuers and health care providers to better facilitate implementation of the most current guidelines into clinical practice [60].

Pertinent changes in the 2015 ACLS guidelines include the addition of an upper limit of 120 compressions per minute [16] resulting from one large registry study that found an association between fast compression rates and inadequate compression depth [61]. Recognizing potential differences in pathophysiologic diseases between shockable and nonshockable initial presenting rhythms leads to differential recommendations with regard to timing of epinephrine administration [58]. The standard dose of 1 mg epinephrine every 3 to 5 minutes remained unchanged, even after treatment of local anesthetic toxicity with Intralipid [62], because no human data to date support a modification in the AHA ACLS recommendations; the latter contrasts with recommendations by other organizations, such as the American Society of Regional Anesthesia and Pain Medicine, which recommend a reduction of epinephrine boluses to less than 1 μg/kg [63]. Epinephrine should be administered as soon as feasible in case of nonshockable compared with shockable rhythms where timely defibrillation remains the treatment of choice. Furthermore, vasopressin has been removed from the algorithm as a vasopressor therapy (see Fig. 1) [16] because of its equivalent effect when compared with epinephrine and the desire to simplify the algorithm. Finally, data indicating that low $ETCO_2$ in intubated patients after 20 minutes of CPR is strongly associated with failure of resuscitation, led to the inclusion of this important parameter as a prognosticator; it should, however, not be used in isolation or in nonintubated patients [16].

New guidelines also exist for the prevention and management of resuscitative emergencies related to opioid and other drug overdoses including local anesthetic systemic toxicity, during the second half of pregnancy, cardiac arrests caused by pulmonary embolism, and those during percutaneous coronary interventions [62].

With regards to mechanical devices, the guidelines have undergone small, but important revisions [64]. Although a clear benefit with the use of automated piston devices versus manual chest compressions has not been found, they provide a reasonable alternative when the delivery of high-quality manual compressions may be challenging or dangerous for the provider, such as with limited personnel, prolonged CPR, in moving ambulances, or during ongoing CPR under fluoroscopy during coronary interventions. In the latter case, the radiolucent backboard of LUCAS seems superior to the one in the AutoPulse device. Furthermore, the combination of an ITD with ACD-CPR was upgraded to a reasonable alternative to conventional CPR when available and used by properly trained personnel [64].

PERIOPERATIVE CONSIDERATIONS

Cardiac arrest during surgery is unique because it is not only witnessed and can be immediately treated, but also because the patient's history is usually well known and vital signs are continuously assessed. Depending on the circumstances, there is a short list of possible causes (see Table 2) that may have led to the perioperative circulatory collapse and that can be treated specifically [11]. Plethysmography or, when available, arterial line traces and $\mathrm{ET}CO_2$ can help assess pulse pressure and rate and cardiac output, respectively; intravenous access and most resuscitative drugs are immediately available in the operating room. All of these allow for a more etiology-specific and immediate management, which largely contributes to an overall higher survival rate [10] than for OHCA and IHCA.

EXPERIMENTAL POSTCONDITIONING TO AMELIORATE GLOBAL ISCHEMIA-REPERFUSION INJURY

Ideally, most patients would receive high-quality CPR by a bystander immediately after cardiac arrest. Unfortunately, in most communities only a minority of patients receives CPR before the arrival of first responders. This translates into an absent circulation with whole-body ischemia for an average of 8 to 10 minutes. In a recent multicenter randomized CPR trial, no patient was discharged from the hospital with favorable neurologic outcome when the time from the emergency call to CPR initiation exceeded 10 minutes [48]. Paradoxically, reperfusion, that is, the reintroduction of blood flow to vital organs after prolonged untreated ischemia, is thought to add significantly to overall ischemia-reperfusion (IR) injury, with mitochondrial dysfunction and the production of reactive oxygen species contributing to cell death [65]. Faced with this challenge, recent research has focused on ways to improve outcomes by mitigating IR injury after cardiac arrest beyond what was previously thought possible. Although preconditioning requires prior knowledge of an ischemic event, postconditioning strategies have the distinct advantage that they can be used on reperfusion [66]. In the context of cardiac arrest, it is important to recognize that the actual reperfusion starts with the onset of CPR, not later with ROSC. Postconditioning is achieved by targeting known intracellular signaling pathways early that lead to cellular dysfunction and eventually cell death. Although its exact signaling mechanisms are still unclear, postconditioning likely includes activation of the reperfusion injury salvage kinase and survival activating factor enhancement pathways, and result in reduced apoptosis and improved cardiac and neurologic function and eventually increased survival in different animal models of cardiac arrest [67]. For example, the introduction of several short well-defined pauses limited to only the very beginning of CPR [68], or the very early administration of pharmacologic agents [69–71] to trigger postconditioning pathways show highly promising results in the experimental setting. Before their translation into clinical practice, however, conclusive clinical trials are needed to understand and validate their benefit in humans.

TARGETED TEMPERATURE MANAGEMENT

The benefits of therapeutic hypothermia to decrease metabolism and thus organ injury following cardiac arrest have been described for several decades [72,73] before the first human trial by Bernard and colleagues [74] in 1997. In 2002, two landmark publications by Bernard and colleagues [75] and the Hypothermia after Cardiac Arrest Study Group [76] built the basis for the current standard of care [77]; therapeutic hypothermia (32°C–34°C) for 18 [75] to 24 hours [76] increased the rate of a favorable neurologic outcome and reduced mortality significantly after cardiac arrest compared with no hypothermia. In 2013, however, Nielsen and colleagues [78] reported in a large multicenter trial that controlled hypothermia did not have any benefit compared with controlled normothermia with regards to mortality or neurologic outcome in unconscious survivors of OHCA. Despite considerable attention and criticism of this study, a possible consensus could be that it may not be the mild hypothermia, but rather the active avoidance of hyperthermia that is critically important for a more favorable outcome post cardiac arrest [78,79]. This notion is now reflected in the 2015 post cardiac arrest care guidelines that now use the new term "targeted temperature management" to refer to induced hypothermia and to the active control of temperature at any target, and recommend that comatose adult patients with ROSC after cardiac arrest are kept at a constant temperature between 32°C and 36°C for at least 24 hours after achieving target temperature [80]. More well-planned studies are necessary to shed more light on this complex topic; underpowered studies [81] with an only presumably negative outcome despite clear evidence to the contrary are of limited usefulness in this context.

SUMMARY

Delivering immediate and high-quality CPR (chest compressions at 100–120 per minute and at least 2 inch deep, full chest recoil, no interruptions, early defibrillation if in a shockable rhythm, no hyperventilation) after cardiac arrest remains the focus of substantial system-based, educational, clinical, and translational research efforts. The high frequency of OHCA and IHCA combined with currently still dismal survival rates lend great significance to any improvement in early restoration of cerebral blood flow and decreasing cerebral IR injury postarrest. Adjunct mechanical devices, such as ACD or automated chest compression devices in combination with an ITD, aim to decrease intrathoracic and intracerebral pressure, thus improving cerebral blood flow and survival; when using an ITD, high-quality CPR is absolutely necessary to benefit the patient. Perioperative cardiac arrest is rare and a special situation because it is typically witnessed and can be treated immediately and specifically according to a short list of likely differential diagnoses. Measuring $ETCO_2$ can add to improve resuscitative efforts, identify ROSC, and contribute to prognostication after prolonged CPR. Postarrest targeted temperature management and, at least in the experimental setting, postconditioning strategies aim to ameliorate cerebral IR injury. Any progress in strengthening one or several links in the chain of survival has the potential to save the lives and to improve the neurologic function of tens of thousands of cardiac arrest patients worldwide each year.

References

[1] Nichol G, Soar J. Regional cardiac resuscitation systems of care. Curr Opin Crit Care 2010;16(3):223–30.
[2] Böttiger BW, Van Aken HK. Saving 100,000 lives each year in Europe. Best Pract Res Clin Anaesthesiol 2013;27(3):291–2.
[3] Nichol G, Thomas E, Callaway CW, et al. Regional variation in out-of-hospital cardiac arrest incidence and outcome. JAMA 2008;300(12):1423–31.
[4] Kleinman ME, Brennan EE, Goldberger ZD, et al. Part 5: adult basic life support and cardiopulmonary resuscitation quality: 2015 American Heart Association guidelines update for cardiopulmonary resuscitation and emergency cardiovascular care. Circulation 2015;132(18 Suppl 2):S414–35.
[5] McNally B, Robb R, Mehta M, et al. Out-of-hospital cardiac arrest surveillance—cardiac arrest registry to enhance survival (CARES), United States, October 1, 2005–December 31, 2010. MMWR Surveill Summ 2011;60(8):1–19.
[6] Sasson C, Rogers MA, Dahl J, et al. Predictors of survival from out-of-hospital cardiac arrest: a systematic review and meta-analysis. Circ Cardiovasc Qual Outcomes 2010;3(1):63–81.
[7] Nolan JP, Soar J, Smith GB, et al. Incidence and outcome of in-hospital cardiac arrest in the United Kingdom National Cardiac Arrest Audit. Resuscitation 2014;85(8):987–92.
[8] Chan PS, Krumholz HM, Spertus JA, et al. Automated external defibrillators and survival after in-hospital cardiac arrest. JAMA 2010;304(19):2129–36.
[9] Fennelly NK, McPhillips C, Gilligan P. Arrest in hospital: a study of in hospital cardiac arrest outcomes. Ir Med J 2014;107(4):105–7.
[10] Ellis SJ, Newland MC, Simonson JA, et al. Anesthesia-related cardiac arrest. Anesthesiology 2014;120(4):829–38.
[11] Moitra VK, Gabrielli A, Maccioli GA, et al. Anesthesia advanced circulatory life support. Can J Anaesth 2012;59(6):586–603.
[12] Safar P. Ventilatory efficacy of mouth-to-mouth artificial respiration; airway obstruction during manual and mouth-to-mouth artificial respiration. J Am Med Assoc 1958;167(3):335–41.
[13] Kouwenhoven WB, Jude JR, Knickerbocker GG. Closed-chest cardiac massage. JAMA 1960;173:1064–7.
[14] Field JM, Hazinski MF, Sayre MR, et al. Part 1: executive summary: 2010 American Heart Association guidelines for cardiopulmonary resuscitation and emergency cardiovascular care. Circulation 2010;122(18 Suppl 3):S640–56.
[15] Lown B, Neuman J, Amarasingham R, et al. Comparison of alternating current with direct electroshock across the closed chest. Am J Cardiol 1962;10:223–33.

[16] Link MS, Berkow LC, Kudenchuk PJ, et al. Part 7: adult advanced cardiovascular life support: 2015 American Heart Association guidelines update for cardiopulmonary resuscitation and emergency cardiovascular care. Circulation 2015;132(18 Suppl 2):S444–64.
[17] Link MS, Atkins DL, Passman RS, et al. Part 6: electrical therapies: automated external defibrillators, defibrillation, cardioversion, and pacing: 2010 American Heart Association guidelines for cardiopulmonary resuscitation and emergency cardiovascular care. Circulation 2010;122(18 Suppl 3):S706–19.
[18] Idris AH, Guffey D, Aufderheide TP, et al. Relationship between chest compression rates and outcomes from cardiac arrest. Circulation 2012;125(24):3004–12.
[19] Edelson DP, Abella BS, Kramer-Johansen J, et al. Effects of compression depth and pre-shock pauses predict defibrillation failure during cardiac arrest. Resuscitation 2006;71(2):137–45.
[20] Hellevuo H, Sainio M, Nevalainen R, et al. Deeper chest compression: more complications for cardiac arrest patients? Resuscitation 2013;84(6):760–5.
[21] Yannopoulos D, McKnite S, Aufderheide TP, et al. Effects of incomplete chest wall decompression during cardiopulmonary resuscitation on coronary and cerebral perfusion pressures in a porcine model of cardiac arrest. Resuscitation 2005;64(3):363–72.
[22] Aufderheide TP, Pirrallo RG, Yannopoulos D, et al. Incomplete chest wall decompression: a clinical evaluation of CPR performance by trained laypersons and an assessment of alternative manual chest compression-decompression techniques. Resuscitation 2006;71(3):341–51.
[23] Fried DA, Leary M, Smith DA, et al. The prevalence of chest compression leaning during in-hospital cardiopulmonary resuscitation. Resuscitation 2011;82(8):1019–24.
[24] Rea TD, Helbock M, Perry S, et al. Increasing use of cardiopulmonary resuscitation during out-of-hospital ventricular fibrillation arrest: survival implications of guideline changes. Circulation 2006;114(25):2760–5.
[25] Aufderheide TP, Sigurdsson G, Pirrallo RG, et al. Hyperventilation-induced hypotension during cardiopulmonary resuscitation. Circulation 2004;109(16):1960–5.
[26] Voorhees WD, Babbs CF, Tacker WA Jr. Regional blood flow during cardiopulmonary resuscitation in dogs. Crit Care Med 1980;8(3):134–6.
[27] Silver DI, Murphy RJ, Babbs CF, et al. Cardiac output during CPR: a comparison of two methods. Crit Care Med 1981;9(5):419–20.
[28] Hightower D, Thomas SH, Stone CK, et al. Decay in quality of closed-chest compressions over time. Ann Emerg Med 1995;26(3):300–3.
[29] Stapleton ER. Comparing CPR during ambulance transport. Manual vs. mechanical methods. JEMS 1991;16(9):63–4, 66, 68 passim.
[30] Lurie KG, Lindo C, Chin J. CPR: the P stands for plumber's helper. JAMA 1990;264(13):1661.
[31] Lurie KG. Active compression-decompression CPR: a progress report. Resuscitation 1994;28(2):115–22.
[32] Cohen TJ, Tucker KJ, Lurie KG, et al. Active compression-decompression. A new method of cardiopulmonary resuscitation. Cardiopulmonary Resuscitation Working Group. JAMA 1992;267(21):2916–23.
[33] Fischer M, Breil M, Ihli M, et al. Mechanical resuscitation assist devices. Anaesthesist 2014;63(3):186–97 [in German].
[34] Halperin HR, Tsitlik JE, Gelfand M, et al. A preliminary study of cardiopulmonary resuscitation by circumferential compression of the chest with use of a pneumatic vest. N Engl J Med 1993;329(11):762–8.
[35] Halperin H, Berger R, Chandra N, et al. Cardiopulmonary resuscitation with a hydraulic-pneumatic band. Crit Care Med 2000;28(11 Suppl):N203–6.
[36] Brooks SC, Toma A, Hsu J. Devices used in cardiac arrest. Emerg Med Clin North Am 2012;30(1):179–93.

[37] Rabl W, Baubin M, Broinger G, et al. Serious complications from active compression-decompression cardiopulmonary resuscitation. Int J Legal Med 1996;109(2):84–9.
[38] Hutchings AC, Darcy KJ, Cumberbatch GL. Tension pneumothorax secondary to automatic mechanical compression decompression device. Emerg Med J 2009;26(2):145–6.
[39] de Rooij PP, Wiendels DR, Snellen JP. Fatal complication secondary to mechanical chest compression device. Resuscitation 2009;80(10):1214–5.
[40] Wind J, Bekkers SC, van Hooren LJ, et al. Extensive injury after use of a mechanical cardiopulmonary resuscitation device. Am J Emerg Med 2009;27(8):1017.e1-2.
[41] Smekal D, Johansson J, Huzevka T, et al. No difference in autopsy detected injuries in cardiac arrest patients treated with manual chest compressions compared with mechanical compressions with the LUCAS device: a pilot study. Resuscitation 2009;80(10):1104–7.
[42] Koster RW, Beenen LF, van der Boom EB, et al. Safety and possible damage from mechanical chest compression during resuscitation. Circulation 2014;130(23):2121–2.
[43] Ochoa FJ, Ramalle-Gomara E, Lisa V, et al. The effect of rescuer fatigue on the quality of chest compressions. Resuscitation 1998;37(3):149–52.
[44] Jones AY, Lee RY. Cardiopulmonary resuscitation and back injury in ambulance officers. Int Arch Occup Environ Health 2005;78(4):332–6.
[45] Keseg DP. The merits of mechanical CPR: do mechanical devices improve compression consistency and resuscitation outcomes? JEMS 2012;37(9):24–9.
[46] Lurie KG, Voelckel WG, Zielinski T, et al. Improving standard cardiopulmonary resuscitation with an inspiratory impedance threshold valve in a porcine model of cardiac arrest. Anesth Analg 2001;93(3):649–55.
[47] Plaisance P, Lurie KG, Payen D. Inspiratory impedance during active compression-decompression cardiopulmonary resuscitation: a randomized evaluation in patients in cardiac arrest. Circulation 2000;101(9):989–94.
[48] Aufderheide TP, Frascone RJ, Wayne MA, et al. Standard cardiopulmonary resuscitation versus active compression-decompression cardiopulmonary resuscitation with augmentation of negative intrathoracic pressure for out-of-hospital cardiac arrest: a randomised trial. Lancet 2011;377(9762):301–11.
[49] Pirrallo RG, Aufderheide TP, Provo TA, et al. Effect of an inspiratory impedance threshold device on hemodynamics during conventional manual cardiopulmonary resuscitation. Resuscitation 2005;66(1):13–20.
[50] Cabrini L, Beccaria P, Landoni G, et al. Impact of impedance threshold devices on cardiopulmonary resuscitation: a systematic review and meta-analysis of randomized controlled studies. Crit Care Med 2008;36(5):1625–32.
[51] Aufderheide TP, Nichol G, Rea TD, et al. A trial of an impedance threshold device in out-of-hospital cardiac arrest. N Engl J Med 2011;365(9):798–806.
[52] Yannopoulos D, Aufderheide TP, Abella BS, et al. Quality of CPR: an important effect modifier in cardiac arrest clinical outcomes and intervention effectiveness trials. Resuscitation 2015;94:106–13.
[53] Yannopoulos D, Nadkarni VM, McKnite SH, et al. Intrathoracic pressure regulator during continuous-chest-compression advanced cardiac resuscitation improves vital organ perfusion pressures in a porcine model of cardiac arrest. Circulation 2005;112(6):803–11.
[54] Yannopoulos D, McKnite S, Metzger A, et al. Intrathoracic pressure regulation improves 24-hour survival in a porcine model of hypovolemic shock. Anesth Analg 2007;104(1):157–62.
[55] Metzger A, Rees J, Kwon Y, et al. Intrathoracic pressure regulation improves cerebral perfusion and cerebral blood flow in a porcine model of brain injury. Shock 2015;44(Suppl 1):96–102.
[56] Huffmyer JL, Groves DS, Scalzo DC, et al. The effect of the intrathoracic pressure regulator on hemodynamics and cardiac output. Shock 2011;35(2):114–6.

[57] Patel N, Branson R, Salter M, et al. "2014 Military supplement" intrathoracic pressure regulation augments stroke volume and ventricular function in human hemorrhage. Shock 2015;44(Suppl 1):55–62.
[58] Neumar RW, Shuster M, Callaway CW, et al. Part 1: executive summary: 2015 American Heart Association guidelines update for cardiopulmonary resuscitation and emergency cardiovascular care. Circulation 2015;132(18 Suppl 2):S315–67.
[59] Kronick SL, Kurz MC, Lin S, et al. Part 4: systems of care and continuous quality improvement: 2015 American Heart Association guidelines update for cardiopulmonary resuscitation and emergency cardiovascular care. Circulation 2015;132(18 Suppl 2):S397–413.
[60] Bhanji F, Donoghue AJ, Wolff MS, et al. Part 14: education: 2015 American Heart Association guidelines update for cardiopulmonary resuscitation and emergency cardiovascular care. Circulation 2015;132(18 Suppl 2):S561–73.
[61] Idris AH, Guffey D, Pepe PE, et al. Chest compression rates and survival following out-of-hospital cardiac arrest. Crit Care Med 2015;43(4):840–8.
[62] Lavonas EJ, Drennan IR, Gabrielli A, et al. Part 10: special circumstances of resuscitation: 2015 American Heart Association guidelines update for cardiopulmonary resuscitation and emergency cardiovascular care. Circulation 2015;132(18 Suppl 2):S501–18.
[63] Neal JM, Bernards CM, Butterworth JF, et al. ASRA practice advisory on local anesthetic systemic toxicity. Reg Anesth Pain Med 2010;35(2):152–61.
[64] Brooks SC, Anderson ML, Bruder E, et al. Part 6: alternative techniques and ancillary devices for cardiopulmonary resuscitation: 2015 American Heart Association guidelines update for cardiopulmonary resuscitation and emergency cardiovascular care. Circulation 2015;132(18 Suppl 2):S436–43.
[65] Kalogeris T, Bao Y, Korthuis RJ. Mitochondrial reactive oxygen species: a double edged sword in ischemia/reperfusion vs preconditioning. Redox Biol 2014;2:702–14.
[66] Hausenloy DJ. Cardioprotection techniques: preconditioning, postconditioning and remote conditioning (basic science). Curr Pharm Des 2013;19(25):4544–63.
[67] Bartos JA, Debaty G, Matsuura T, et al. Post-conditioning to improve cardiopulmonary resuscitation. Curr Opin Crit Care 2014;20(3):242–9.
[68] Segal N, Matsuura T, Caldwell E, et al. Ischemic postconditioning at the initiation of cardiopulmonary resuscitation facilitates functional cardiac and cerebral recovery after prolonged untreated ventricular fibrillation. Resuscitation 2012;83(11):1397–403.
[69] Meybohm P, Gruenewald M, Albrecht M, et al. Pharmacological postconditioning with sevoflurane after cardiopulmonary resuscitation reduces myocardial dysfunction. Crit Care 2011;15(5):R241.
[70] Riess ML, Matsuura TR, Bartos JA, et al. Anaesthetic postconditioning at the initiation of CPR improves myocardial and mitochondrial function in a Pig model of prolonged untreated ventricular fibrillation. Resuscitation 2014;85(12):1745–51.
[71] Bartos JA, Matsuura TR, Sarraf M, et al. Bundled postconditioning therapies improve hemodynamics and neurologic recovery after 17 min of untreated cardiac arrest. Resuscitation 2015;87:7–13.
[72] Benson DW, Williams GR Jr, Spencer FC, et al. The use of hypothermia after cardiac arrest. Anesth Analg 1959;38:423–8.
[73] Safar P, Xiao F, Radovsky A, et al. Improved cerebral resuscitation from cardiac arrest in dogs with mild hypothermia plus blood flow promotion. Stroke 1996;27(1):105–13.
[74] Bernard SA, Jones BM, Horne MK. Clinical trial of induced hypothermia in comatose survivors of out-of-hospital cardiac arrest. Ann Emerg Med 1997;30(2):146–53.
[75] Bernard SA, Gray TW, Buist MD, et al. Treatment of comatose survivors of out-of-hospital cardiac arrest with induced hypothermia. N Engl J Med 2002;346(8):557–63.
[76] Hypothermia after Cardiac Arrest Study Group. Mild therapeutic hypothermia to improve the neurologic outcome after cardiac arrest. N Engl J Med 2002;346(8):549–56.

[77] Peberdy MA, Callaway CW, Neumar RW, et al. Part 9: post-cardiac arrest care: 2010 American Heart Association guidelines for cardiopulmonary resuscitation and emergency cardiovascular care. Circulation 2010;122(18 Suppl 3):S768–86.
[78] Nielsen N, Wetterslev J, Cronberg T, et al. Targeted temperature management at 33 degrees C versus 36 degrees C after cardiac arrest. N Engl J Med 2013;369(23):2197–206.
[79] Little NE, Feldman EL. Therapeutic hypothermia after cardiac arrest without return of consciousness: skating on thin ice. JAMA Neurol 2014;71(7):823–4.
[80] Callaway CW, Donnino MW, Fink EL, et al. Part 8: post-cardiac arrest care: 2015 American Heart Association guidelines update for cardiopulmonary resuscitation and emergency cardiovascular care. Circulation 2015;132(18 Suppl 2):S465–82.
[81] Moler FW, Silverstein FS, Holubkov R, et al. Therapeutic hypothermia after out-of-hospital cardiac arrest in children. N Engl J Med 2015;372(20):1898–908.

Advances in Anesthesia 34 (2016) 47–61

ADVANCES IN ANESTHESIA

Environmental Sustainability in Anesthesia

Pollution Prevention and Patient Safety

Jodi Sherman, MD[a,*], Forbes McGain, FANZCA, FCICM[b]

[a]Department of Anesthesiology, Yale University, School of Medicine, 333 Cedar Street, TMP3, New Haven, CT 06520, USA; [b]Departments of Anaesthesia and Intensive Care, Western Health, Gordon Street, Footscray, Victoria 3054, Australia

Keywords

• Anesthesia • Ecologocial sustainability • Pollution prevention • Patient safety
• Life cycle assessment • Environmental engineering

Key points

- Health care pollution is a hidden patient safety issue. In 2013, the US health care sector contributed nearly 10% of the nation's greenhouse gas (GHG) emissions.
- Anesthesiology is a resource-intense specialty, providing opportunities for leadership to reduce health care pollution. Inhaled anesthetics are potent GHG, accounting for 2.5% of the UK's health sector GHG emissions.
- Many strategies are immediately available for reduction of waste and pollution from operating rooms and perioperative areas.
- The environmental sustainability of anesthetic practice varies considerably between nations, even without differences in patient outcomes. Exploration of why this occurs could be financially and environmentally rewarding.
- The research base of hospital sustainability is at an early stage; considerable opportunities lie ahead.

> Do the best you can until you know better. Then when you know better, do better.
>
> —Maya Angelou

Disclosure: Dr J. Sherman has no financial relationships with industry. Dr J. Sherman is supported by a grant from the Anesthesia Patient Safety Foundation. Dr F. McGain has no financial relationships with industry.

*Corresponding author. *E-mail address:* jodi.sherman@yale.edu

http://dx.doi.org/10.1016/j.aan.2016.07.004

INTRODUCTION

Health care pollution is a hidden patient safety issue that can no longer be ignored. The US health sector presently accounts for 17% of national gross domestic product, and is highly interconnected with industrial activities that significantly contribute to national emissions to air, water, and land. In 2013, the US health care sector contributed nearly 10% of the nation's greenhouse gas (GHG) emissions [1,2]. If the US health sector were a country itself, it would rank 13th in the world for GHG emissions. These emissions stem from the entire life cycle of products and services ("cradle to grave"), including direct care and purchases (46%), as well as indirect supply chain activities (54%). Similar reporting from the United Kingdom noted that, of the National Health Service (NHS) GHG emissions, 22% stemmed from pharmaceuticals (excluding waste anesthetic gas) and 13% from medical devices [3,4]. Inhaled anesthetics alone accounted for 2.5% of the entire NHS health sector GHG emissions [5]. Environmental health is linked critically to human health, and because anesthesiology is a resource-intense specialty, there is much that anesthesiologists can do to lessen the disease burden that stems from clinical care itself. If the current trajectory of modern medicine is left unmitigated, the costs of "business as usual" will contribute to the worsening of public health and an increase in the demand for health services. Anesthesiologists have both an opportunity for and obligation to pollution prevention, to protect patients and society.

Climate change

The World Health Organization named climate change the defining issue for health systems in the 21st century [6]. The United Nations Framework Convention on Climate Change recognizes 6 disease categories linked to climate change: cardiovascular disease, asthma and respiratory disease, infectious disease, compromised food and water security, increased weather disturbances, and threat to blood supply through changing vectors for blood borne illnesses [7]. Currently, an estimated 150,000 patients die annually in the world owing to climate change–related disease, and if left unchecked a predicted 500,000 will die per year by 2050 [2]. The World Health Organization calls on physicians to use their authority to lead mitigation, and protect public health [6]. Although GHG are a critical category of emissions that threaten human health and society [6], there are several other categories of environmental pollution important to consider.

Chemical pollution

Each year, the US produces or imports nearly 860 million tons of chemicals [8–10]. Pharmaceutical and industrial chemical pollutants have become widespread in the environment and food chains, and are also found in humans. Unlike pharmaceuticals, current regulation of industrial chemicals in the United States is covered under the Toxic Substance Control Act of 1976 and does not require safety testing before introduction into the marketplace. The Centers for Disease Control and Prevention only recently began providing an ongoing assessment of the exposure of the US population to environmental chemicals through biomonitoring [11]. Of the approximately 100,000 industrial chemicals in the marketplace, only about 400 are currently looked for in humans and, of those, hundreds of pollutants can be routinely found in any human being. Contamination of humans by hundreds of synthetic chemicals has been documented, and observed in amniotic fluid [12], in cord blood at birth [13], as well as adults [11]. Many of these substances are known carcinogens, teratogens, neurodevelopmental toxicants, and endocrine disruptors [14,15]. An estimated 12.3 million deaths–nearly one-quarter of all deaths worldwide–every year are owing to unhealthy environments [16]. Although practitioners do not typically think about how clinical care places demands on industry, it is important to recognize that the health sector is the second largest chemical purchaser in the United States. [8–10].

QUANTIFYING ENVIRONMENTAL AND HUMAN HEALTH IMPACTS FROM POLLUTION: LIFE CYCLE ASSESSMENT

To guide mitigation strategies in patient care, clinical pollution requires quantification. Life cycle assessment (LCA) is an internationally accepted scientific method to quantify emissions and multiple environmental and public health impacts of a product or process over its entire life span. The total life cycle ("cradle to grave") includes natural resource extraction, device manufacturing, transport, use/reuse, and disposal. In this way, LCA accounts for direct and indirect emissions, including upstream and downstream impacts, to help identify hotspots for targeted improvement efforts and informed decision making. Guidance documents have been promulgated by the US Environmental Protection Agency, the Society for Environmental Toxicologists and Chemists, and standards have been issued by the International Organization of Standardization 14,040 series [17–20].

LCA illuminates particular processes or substances that contribute significantly to impacts, and enables comparison of related products along environmental dimensions. Several standard LCA impact categories exist, including GHG emissions (carbon dioxide equivalents [CO_2e]) contributing to climate change; stratospheric ozone depletion; respiratory disease from inhalation of particulate matter and ground-level ozone (smog); cancer and noncancer disease owing to chemical exposure; acidification and eutrophication (excess nutrients leading to algae blooms) in soils and surface waters; and ecotoxicity chemical burden on aquatic organism ecosystems. CO2e emissions are the most commonly reported impact category; however, LCA may demonstrate comparative advantages or disadvantages in various categories, and prioritization of risks and benefits must be weighted as other types of pollutants may be more and others less favorable [1].

LCA is commonly used in different sectors, from chemicals to consumer products to systems, to compare options and identify opportunities for design and utilization improvements. Applications to health care are relatively new, and beginning to gain foothold to guide pollution prevention strategies. LCA applications to health care have included hemodialysis practices [21], nonsurgical management approaches to acute myocardial infarction [22], management of labor and delivery [23], and surgical approaches to hysterectomy [24]. LCA applications to anesthetic drugs and devices are also appearing, and can aid anesthesiologists in decision making [25–28]. In 2012, the UK NHS launched the GHG *Protocol Product Life Cycle Accounting and Reporting Standard* project, to encompass the pharmaceutical and medical device sector [29]. The goal is for all drugs and devices to undergo LCA, to guide routine health systems improvement.

INHALED ANESTHETICS AND ATMOSPHERIC POLLUTION

Inhaled anesthetics are potent GHGs. These drugs undergo very little in vivo metabolism, and are exhaled virtually unconsumed and unchanged into anesthesia machines or the indoor atmosphere. Exhaled agents are "scavenged" by anesthesia machines and then vented directly into the atmosphere as medical waste gases. All exhaled anesthetic gases remain for extended periods in the troposphere–the lowest layer of the atmosphere in which the greenhouse effect occurs: sevoflurane for 1.1 years, isoflurane for 3.2 years, desflurane for 14 years, and nitrous oxide for 114 years. Global warming potential (GWP) is a measure of the ability to trap heat, and is determined by the atmospheric lifetime of a gas combined with its infrared absorption property. Carbon dioxide (CO_2) serves as the reference point, with a GWP = 1. Other substances are converted into CO_2e, enabling comparisons over a given time period. A GWP 100-year (GWP_{100}) time frame is commonly reported in the international community. GWP_{100} for anesthetic gases include: sevoflurane for 130, isoflurane for 510, desflurane for 2540, and nitrous oxide for 298 [30].

In addition to GWPs, drug potency and fresh gas flow rates must be considered for meaningful comparisons between anesthetic gases [31]. When a steady-state hourly amount of anesthetic necessary for 1 minimum alveolar concentration (MAC) at 2 liters per minute (LPM) for sevoflurane, and 1 LPM for desflurane and isoflurane is weighted by the GWP, the clinically relevant quantities of each anesthetic can then be compared. On a per-MAC-hour basis, the total life cycle GHG impact of desflurane is more than 20 times higher than isoflurane and sevoflurane. Because of nitrous oxide's low potency and therefore high concentration requirements, and its long atmospheric lifetime, its GHG impacts are similar to desflurane on a per-MAC-hour basis. When used as a carrier, nitrous oxide dramatically worsens the GHG emissions profiles of sevoflurane and isoflurane. All inhaled drugs are potent GHGs in and of themselves, and the waste phase dominates the life cycle impacts. By comparison, the total life cycle GHG effects of propofol are quite small, nearly 4 orders of magnitude lower than those of desflurane or nitrous oxide. Propofol's GHG impacts (including plastic syringe, tubing, and packaging) primarily stem from the use phase owing to electricity requirements for pump delivery systems [25].

Inhaled anesthetics and the operating room footprint

The life cycle GHG emissions of 4 different surgical approaches to hysterectomy have recently been analyzed in the United States [24]. The average GHG emissions of 62 hysterectomies varied based on the surgical approach. Abdominal and vaginal hysterectomies showed similar trends, with average GHG emissions approximately one-half as high as laparoscopic approaches and one-third as high as when robotic techniques were used, predominantly owing to fewer disposable instruments and linens. The average GHG impacts of anesthetic gases accounted for approximately 70% of the emissions for abdominal and vaginal surgical approaches, and 30% for laparoscopic and robotic approaches. Inhaled anesthetics thus dominated the combined surgical and anesthetic total GHG footprint, even when taking into account the energy requirements for the heating, ventilation, and air conditioning system and electrical equipment.

National contributions of inhaled anesthetics

The UK Sustainability Development Unit reported that their health sector is responsible for 3% to 4% of their national GHG [3]. Inhaled anesthetics accounted for 2.5% of the entire UK health sector GHG emissions [5]. The US health sector contributes an estimated 10% of national GHG [1]. US impacts from inhaled anesthetics were estimated at 5.6 million metric tons or 1% of US national GHGs (excluding dental, laboratory, and veterinary medicine) [32].

Global contributions of inhaled anesthetics

Sulbaek Anderson and colleagues [33,34] have estimated the total worldwide contribution of inhaled anesthetics to global warming at 0.01% (excluding dental, laboratory and veterinary medicine). This estimate is cited commonly as a reason to neglect pollution prevention by anesthesiologists; however, such a conclusion is problematic. This estimate is extrapolated from only 1 US institution's anesthetic practices, and this institution used virtually no desflurane. Researchers neglected to include nitrous oxide in their calculations, and reported an erroneous average of 17 kg CO_2e per anesthetic. However, institutions that use some desflurane and account for nitrous oxide have reported an average of 175 to 220 kg CO_2e per anesthetic [32]. Sulbaek-Anderson's group [34] therefore likely substantially underestimated the total worldwide contribution of inhaled anesthetics.

Vollmer and colleagues [35] recently reported actual measurements of atmospheric concentrations of volatile anesthetics. Nitrous oxide was excluded owing to its multiple sources beyond health care. Researchers sampled different urban areas and Antarctica from 2004 to 2014, and detected "a rapid accumulation and ubiquitous presence of isoflurane, desflurane, and sevoflurane in the global atmosphere." The calculated global combined release to the atmosphere of volatile anesthetic gases was 3.1 ± 0.6 million metric tons CO_2e in 2014, of which approximately 80% stemmed from desflurane. This is equivalent to the CO_2 emissions of approximately 650,000 passenger vehicles.

Ozone depletion

Separate from GHG effects, nitrous oxide, and to a lesser extent halothane, are destructive to the ozone layer. The ozone layer serves to protect the Earth from ultraviolet radiation, and its destruction leaves humans and other animals more vulnerable to skin cancers. Nitrous oxide emissions are the single most important threat to the ozone layer, and anthropogenic emissions represent the largest source [36]. Most N_2O emissions come from fertilizer for industrial agriculture; however, medical use is also significant. N_2O seems to be gaining in popularity, particularly in birthing suites where it is delivered at high fresh gas flows. As with all inhaled anesthetics, N_2O is ultimately vented directly to the atmosphere virtually unchanged, where it persists the longest of all the medical gases (114 years).

SOLUTIONS: INHALED ANESTHETIC POLLUTION PREVENTION

Lowest fresh gas flows

Conscious effort should be made to minimize fresh gas flows [32,37,38]. After induction and before intubation, turning off fresh gas flows, as opposed to the more common practice of turning off the vaporizer, prevents waste and flushing of the system into the indoor environment. Avoiding unnecessary flushing of the circuit prevents excess occupational exposure and maintains drug concentration in the system. Attention should be made to reducing fresh gas flows immediately after the induction sequence is complete. Low maintenance flows should be chosen: 1 LPM for sevoflurane up to 2-MAC-hours, then 2 LPM in the United States; for desflurane and isoflurane, less than 1 LPM can be maintained. High fresh gas flows for emergence are ideally reserved until the vaporizers are turned off. High fresh gas flows should never be used as a method to cool patients, because it is highly inefficient compared with other solutions. High fresh gas flows ought to be conscientiously reserved for quick changes in anesthetic depth only.

Anesthetic choice

Clinical circumstances dictate the indicated anesthetic. Where choices exist in how to safely administer care, as they often do, pollution prevention ought to weigh into clinical decision-making to protect public health [32]. Environmental research suggests that desflurane and nitrous oxide should be reserved for only those cases where they could reduce morbidity and mortality over other drug combinations. These inhaled anesthetics have lower solubility, and therefore faster emergence profiles for short cases compared with drugs with greater solubility. However, with a little practice, the timing of emergence for any drug, even those with greater solubility, can be mastered. Nitrous oxide should not be used simply to spare volatile anesthetics, such as during the emergence phase. N_2O for routine labor analgesia ought to be reconsidered where alternatives exist. When clinically appropriate, intravenous anesthesia and regional anesthesia techniques often provide the most environmentally sound approaches.

Waste anesthetic gas capture versus destruction

Waste anesthetic gas capturing technologies prevent waste anesthetic gas release into the environment, and reclaim the drug for potential reseparation and reuse. One type of waste anesthetic gas capturing can be built or retrofitted into the exhaust system of the operating room and is activated only when the patient exhales, as opposed to standard continuous vacuuming systems (thereby saving considerable energy use) [39]. Another system requires simple installation of a canister into existing scavenging circuits, adsorbs the volatile anesthetic drugs, and the canister is either discarded (approximately once per week, depending on use patterns) or stored [40]. Neither system captures N_2O, however. Application has been made to the US Food and Drug Administration for approval to reuse reclaimed volatile drugs, which could also find applications in laboratory and veterinary medicine. Technologies on the near horizon include photochemical air purification, which can destroy (but not capture for reuse) all waste anesthetic gas, including N_2O.

PHARMACEUTICAL POLLUTION

In the United Kingdom, the NHS reported 22% of its health sector GHG footprint stemmed from pharmaceuticals (excluding waste anesthetic gas) [3]. Manufacturing contributed the greatest amount of all the life cycle phases, suggesting the importance of improved efficiency for both industry and clinical practices.

In addition to GHGs, chemical pollution is concerning. The majority of all medications ingested are secreted in the urine, either unchanged or as metabolites. Medications are often adapted to resist biodegradation and can therefore remain in the environment for a long time. Municipal wastewater treatment currently does not process drugs. Many medications have been found in drinking water, indicating that current handling is inadequate. Small amounts and unknown synergies may result in developmental disorders where timing of exposure is critical.

SOLUTIONS: PHARMACEUTICAL POLLUTION PREVENTION

Drug choices and manufacturing

There is little information available to health care providers that adequately compares or standardizes the environmental harm of pharmaceuticals. The environmental department of the Stockholm County Council [41] initiated an environmental hazard assessment in 2003, aimed at reducing pharmaceutical residues in the ground, water, and air. A hazard "PBT" Index for substances emerged that newly includes persistence (P) and bioaccumulation (B), in addition to traditional consideration for toxicity (T). When choices exist, the PBT index is intended to aid clinicians in giving priority to pharmaceuticals that are least harmful to the environment. Only some anesthesia drugs have been indexed thus far. In 2012, the UK NHS launched the *Greenhouse Gas Protocol Product Life Cycle Accounting and Reporting Standard* project, to encompass the pharmaceutical and medical device sector [29]. The NHS project in the near future will aid clinicians in, and direct industry toward, environmentally safer practices, however it currently focuses only on greenhouse gas emissions.

Reduce pharmaceutical waste

In addition to selecting and developing low-impact pharmaceuticals, it is critical to prevent pharmaceutical waste. The use of prepackaged drug syringes (third-party vendor or in house) is gaining in popularity to increase shelf-life and reduce waste. Single-use vials are often too large for a single patient [42,43] and newer regulations in the US limit the ability to split drugs from multiuse vials, costing billions of dollars in waste [42]. Waste prevention entices drug splitting by anesthesia staff, despite regulations against such practice to prevent cross-contamination. It is therefore a patient safety issue to use hospital pharmacy services to divide doses, even for cheaper drugs. Beyond prefilled syringes, clinicians ought to always select the smallest vials/ampoules feasible. Effort should be made to predict the duration of cases, levels of stimulation, and patient tolerances to aid in estimating drug requirements. If the most appropriate size vial is not conveniently located, effort should be made to contact pharmacy to address systems improvement.

Proper pharmaceutical waste disposal

Every effort should be made to avoid wasting drugs into wastewater drains, or into the regular trash, which becomes destined for landfill. Drugs ought to be wasted into the appropriate bin. Acutely toxic "P-listed" drugs (eg, epinephrine and nitroglycerin) typically go in a black bin, and require the most costly and energy-intensive processing (high heat incineration.) The vast majority of anesthetic drugs may go into the "non-RCRC" (The Resource Conservation and Recovery Act) bin, typically "purple" or "purple/white," also destined for incineration (at a lower temperature.) Dedicated waste bins are always preferable to dumping down the drain, as is common practice in the United States, to avoid diversion of opioids. Opioids may be managed by using bins with stabilizers so they are "nonreclaimable," and then instead discarded either to landfills or incinerated. Propofol should be managed through incineration only, as is recommended by the manufacturer. Propofol is toxic to ecosystems and should not be discarded to wastewater drains or to regular trash.

REUSABLE VERSUS SINGLE-USE DISPOSABLE MEDICAL DEVICES

Criteria for the selection and purchase of medical devices typically include safety for patients and staff, efficacy and ease of use, and purchase and handling costs. On the basis of such criteria, single-use disposable medical devices are increasingly supplanting reusable devices in the United States and elsewhere [8]. In the United Kingdom, 13% of the national health sector GHG footprint stems from medical devices [3,4]. The increase in disposables is largely attributed to infection prevention, however without much supporting evidence of superiority over proper cleaning of reusable devices. US hospitals now throw away 5.9 million tons of hospital waste per year [44].

Problems with plastic

Plastic can last hundreds of years in the environment. Incinerating plastic produces many harmful chemicals such as heavy metals, air pollutants, and carcinogens including dioxin. In 1996, the US Environmental Protection Agency declared medical waste incineration the number 1 source of dioxin contamination in the atmosphere. This declaration lead to a Memorandum of Understanding between the US Environmental Protection Agency and the American Hospitals Association [45], resulting in the closure of the majority of medical incinerators. Regular medical waste is now largely treated and sent to landfills; however, this trend is reversing as landfills are maxing out and "waste-to-energy" incineration is increasing. Proper attention to correct waste segregation is essential to minimize unnecessary incineration, save money, and prevent pollution.

SOLUTIONS: SOLID WASTE STREAM DIVERSION: REUSING, REPROCESSING, AND RECYCLING

Reusables versus disposables

Purchase and maintenance costs for disposable devices are typically perceived to be less than for reusables, yet in reality expenses are spread across multiple cost centers making comprehensive assessment challenging. LCA includes manufacturing, materials, labor, and energy and water use on the front end and disposal labor, landfill, and incineration costs on the back end. Economic costs and environmental impacts often favor reusable equipment [26,46,47].

Laryngeal mask airways provide a good anesthesia example. The purchase of disposable laryngeal mask airways is frequently believed less expensive. A recent LCA comparing reusable and disposable laryngeal mask airways found that reusable masks were environmentally preferable to disposables if used at least 10 times, and more cost effective if used at least 20 times at a large urban US hospital (one-half of the manufacturer-rated lifetime, with reports of more than 100 uses in the literature) [26]. For both environmental and economic considerations, management and operating procedures should ensure that reusable equipment is not discarded prematurely. These benefits must be weighed against concerns regarding transmission of infection, although routine use of disposables seems to be unwarranted [26].

Reprocessing of single-use devices

Another option that can lower environmental impact of disposable items is the reprocessing of single-use items through a third-party vendor. Medical devices sold as "single use," are designated as such by the manufacturer, and not the US Food and Drug Administration. Several companies now reprocess these used equipment items. Equipment is collected, cleaned, tested to ensure performance mandated by the US Food and Drug Administration [48], then resterilized and repackaged, and resold and tracked for a limited number of reprocessings. Unlike new items that are sample batch tested, every reprocessed device is tested, and a US Government Accountability Office investigation demonstrated that device failure rate is no different between new and reprocessed items [49]. In addition to waste stream diversion, reprocessed items may be sold back to hospitals with as much as a 50% discount. Surgical and anesthetic devices such as laparoscopic trocars, pulse oximeter probes, blood pressure cuffs, and laryngoscope blades and handles can be reprocessed routinely. Reprocessing reduces environmental impacts of de novo manufacturing, and provides considerable cost savings on disposal and purchasing [50].

Clinical recycling

Recycling is now making its way into ORs. *Without doubt, reduction of waste and reuse of devices are preferable to recycling.* When these are not possible, significant cost and environmental savings can be achieved through waste stream diversion with recycling. OR recycling may be achieved through collecting items during case setup, before a patient is brought into the room, when more than one third of OR waste is generated. Doing so before bringing patients into the OR reduces risk of contamination of recycling waste by potentially infectious material. This is a common strategy to prevent cross contamination in new clinical recycling programs, and ought to be used at least until staff are educated on proper waste segregation. Single-source waste stream recycling (ie, placing different plastics, cardboard and alumina in the one bin) is gaining in popularity, making collection simple by eliminating the need to separate types of materials [51,52].

THE INTERNATIONAL PERSPECTIVE

Considerable differences exist in the anesthetic drug and equipment management seen in different nations, even between countries with similar socioeconomic standing. The choice of anesthetic agent can vary markedly. For example, a 2011 survey of Scandinavian anesthesiologists showed that N_2O was used in Denmark in only 0.6% of general anesthetics versus 39% in Iceland. More surprising, only 22% of general anesthetics involved the use of volatile agents in Denmark, contrasting with 92% in Iceland [53]. The predominant use of intravenous anesthesia in Denmark was only partly attributable to environmental concerns, but indicates an environmental awareness among some anesthesiologists. The use of sevoflurane with low fresh gas flows is not recommended by the US Food and Drug Administration, nor the equivalent UK and Australian regulatory agencies, despite randomized controlled evidence to the contrary [54]. Nevertheless, anecdotally, many UK and Australian anesthesiologists use low-flow (1 L/min or less) sevoflurane in contrast with their US colleagues, without evidence of ill effect.

In the operating room in the United States, the majority of devices used are now single-use, including pulse oximeters, blood pressure cuffs, breathing circuits, and facemasks. The United States seems to be leading the way in reprocessing medical equipment, perhaps because the single-use market is so expansive. However, reprocessing still diverts only a small amount of single-use disposables from the waste stream. In Australia, the United Kingdom, and elsewhere, single-use disposable pulse oximeters and blood pressure cuffs are almost unheard of. Anesthetic breathing circuits are single use in the United

Box 1: ASA Anesthesiology sustainability checklist

1. Reduce inhaled anesthetic atmospheric waste.
   a. Use low fresh gas flows.
   b. Avoid high impact inhaled anesthetics: desflurane, nitrous oxide.
   c. Consider intravenous and regional techniques.
   d. Invest in WAG trapping (for volatiles only) or WAG destroying (all inhaled anesthetics, including Nitrous Oxide) technology for the Anesthesia Machine.
2. Reduce intravenous pharmaceutical waste.
   a. Use prefilled syringes.
   b. Use appropriate sized vials for an individual patient.
   c. Dispose of unused medications and vials according to regulations.
3. Reduce anesthesia equipment waste.
   a. Only open equipment intended for immediate use.
   b. Consider purchase of reusable or reprocessed equipment over disposable.
   c. Reprocess or recycle suitable disposable equipment.
   d. Adjust stock levels to minimize discarding expired items.
   e. Reformulate prefabricated kits to eliminate unnecessary items.
   f. Reformulate anesthesia supply carts to eliminate unnecessary items.
   g. Donate expired or unused open equipment.
4. Solid waste segregation
   a. Segregate waste according to type (pharmaceutical, solid, biohazard, etc).
   b. Avoid default of placing all solid waste into biohazard or sharps bins.
   c. Recycle batteries.
   d. Consider intraoperative recycling program for clean plastics, paper and cardboard.
   e. Use reusable sharps containers.
5. Linens
   a. Consider reusable linens.
   b. Minimize excessive use of reusable and disposable cotton towels and blankets.
6. Electronics
   a. Avoid excess electronics without proven benefit to patient care.
   b. Use a certified sustainable electronics recycling vendor to dispose of old equipment.
   c. When negotiating equipment upgrades, request vendors take back old equipment and refurbish to donate, or request vendor use a certified sustainable electronics recycling vendor.

7. Leadership
   a. Develop/join a sustainability committee at a department, hospital, or society level and advocate for a sustainability officer.
   b. Collaborate with the hospital sustainability officer to embed sustainability as part of 'core business', improving public health for the surrounding community, and 'first do no harm.'
   c. Become involved in environmental preferable purchasing.
   d. Educate staff regarding the health, safety, and cost benefits of environmental projects.
   e. Evaluate new equipment, facility, and behavior options for improved sustainability.
   f. Consider strategic sustainability research projects that will lead to financial and environmental savings for the hospital.

From the American Society of Anesthesiologists Environmental Task Force, 'Greening the Operating Room and Perioperative Arena'. Available at: http://www.asahq.org/resources/resources-from-asa-committees/greening-the-operating-room. Accessed March 28, 2016.

States, differing markedly with the approach in Europe [55], Australia [56], and elsewhere. Facemasks, surgical gowns, and theater packs are routinely single use in the United States, but often reusable in many countries. The reasons for such differences in the use of reusable and single-use disposable equipment are multifactorial, and include perceptions around financial, cultural, legislative, and infection control concerns. The significance of any advantages to patient safety are largely unproven, and secondary disease burden through pollution is a neglected issue.

SUMMARY: ENVIRONMENTAL IMPACT AND ANESTHESIA PRACTICE

The ecological footprint of health care is enormous. Noble concern and care for the individual patient often neglects the impact of such dedicated practice on community and planetary health. The ecological footprint of perioperative practice is one of the largest in all of health care, representing more than one-third of all hospital resources and waste. Exploration of why there is such variability in the environmental footprint of anesthetic practice in different countries, without evidence in differing outcomes, would be worthwhile. Many strategies are immediately available for reduction of waste and pollution from operating rooms and perioperative areas (Box 1). These include environmentally preferable purchasing, shifting back to more common use of reusable devices, reprocessing equipment, recycling materials, donating equipment to programs such as REMEDY [50], and energy efficient redesign of the operating room [57]. Additionally, clinicians can select "least-impact" drugs [25], use prepackaged syringes, minimize fresh gas flows, and use intravenous anesthesia and regional anesthesia when safe and feasible. Education and awareness may be the greatest barriers to broad implementation [58,59].

References

[1] Eckelman M, Sherman J. Environmental impacts of the U.S. health care system and effects on public health. PLoS One 2016;11(6):e0157014.

[2] Mis M. Climate change impact predicted to cause 500,000 deaths in 2050. Available at: http://www.reuters.com/article/us-health-climatechange-food-idUSKCN0W503S. Accessed March 28, 2016.

[3] Sustainable Development Unit. NHS England Carbon Footprint 2012. London (England): National Health Service; 2012.

[4] Sustainable Development Unit. Goods and Services Carbon Hotspots. London (England): National Health Service; 2012.

[5] Sustainable Development Unit. Carbon footprint from anaesthetic gas use 2013. London (England): National Health Service; 2013.

[6] Chan M. World Health Organization: Protecting health from climate change. Available at: http://whqlibdoc.who.int/publications/2009/9789241598880_eng.pdf. Accessed March 28, 2016.

[7] World Health Organization (WHO) IPCC. Climate change 2007: Impacts, Adaptation, and Vulnerability–Contribution of Working Group II to the Fourth Assessment Report of the Intergovernmental Panel on Climate Change. Available at: http://www.ipcc-wg2.org/index.html. Accessed March 28, 2016.

[8] Sherman JD, Ryan S. Ecological responsibility in anesthesia practice. Int Anesthesiol Clin 2010;48:139–51.

[9] American Chemistry Council. The business of chemistry: by the numbers. Available at: https://www.americanchemistry.com/chemistry-industry-facts. Accessed March 28, 2016.

[10] American Chemistry Council. U.S. Business of Chemistry Flow Chart. Available at: https://www.americanchemistry.com/Jobs/EconomicStatistics/Chemistry-in-Economy/Chemistry-Dependent-Economy/US-Business-of-Chemistry-Flow-Chart.html. Accessed March 28, 2016.

[11] Centers for Disease Control and Prevention (CDC). CDC National Biomonitoring Program. Available at: http://www.cdc.gov/biomonitoring/. Accessed March 28, 2016.

[12] Jensen MS, Norgaard-Pedersen B, Toft G, et al. Phthalates and perfluorooctanesulfonic acid in human amniotic fluid: temporal trends and timing of amniocentesis in pregnancy. Environ Health Perspect 2012;120:897–903.

[13] Environmental Working Group (EWG). Pollution in Minority Newborns. Available at: http://www.ewg.org/research/minority-cord-blood-report/executive-summary. Accessed March 28, 2016.

[14] Collaborative on Health and the Environment. Consensus Statement. Available at: http://www.healthandenvironment.org/about/consensus. Accessed March 28, 2016.

[15] Centers for Disease Control and Prevention (CDC). National Report on Human Exposure to Environmental Chemicals. Available at: http://www.cdc.gov/exposurereport/. Accessed March 28, 2016.

[16] Pruss-Ustun AWJ, Corvalan C, Bos R, et al. Preventing Disease through Healthy Environments: a global assessment of the burden of disease from environmental risks. Geneva (Switzerland): World Health Organization; 2016.

[17] International Organization for Standardization. ISO 14044:2006 Environmental management–Life cycle assessment–requirements and guidelines. Available at: http://www.iso.org/iso/catalogue_detail?csnumber=38498. Accessed March 28, 2016.

[18] Vigon W, Tolle D. Life cycle assessment: inventory guidelines and principles. Cincinnati (OH): Battelle and Franklin Associates; 1992.

[19] UNEP/SETAC. Life cycle approaches: the road from analysis to practice. Paris (France): UNEP/SETAC; 2005.

[20] Fava J, Denison R, Jones B, et al. A technical framework for life cycle assessment. Washington, DC: SETAC and SETAC Foundation for Environmental Education, Inc.; 1991.

[21] Connor A, Lillywhite R, Cooke MW. The carbon footprints of home and in-center maintenance hemodialysis in the United Kingdom. Hemodial Int 2011;15:39–51.
[22] Zander A, Niggebrugge A, Pencheon D, et al. Changes in travel-related carbon emissions associated with modernization of services for patients with acute myocardial infarction: a case study. J Public Health (Oxf) 2011;33:272–9.
[23] Campion N, Thiel CL, DeBlois J, et al. Life cycle assessment perspectives on delivering an infant in the US. Sci Total Environ 2012;425:191–8.
[24] Thiel CL, Eckelman M, Guido R, et al. Environmental impacts of surgical procedures: life cycle assessment of hysterectomy in the United States. Environ Sci Technol 2015;49:1779–86.
[25] Sherman J, Le C, Lamers V, et al. Life cycle greenhouse gas emissions of anesthetic drugs. Anesth Analg 2012;114:1086–90.
[26] Eckelman M, Mosher M, Gonzalez A, et al. Comparative life cycle assessment of disposable and reusable laryngeal mask airways. Anesth Analg 2012;114:1067–72.
[27] McGain F, Story D, Kayak E, et al. Workplace sustainability: the "cradle to grave" view of what we do. Anesth Analg 2012;114:1134–9.
[28] McGain F, McAlister S, McGavin A, et al. A life cycle assessment of reusable and single-use central venous catheter insertion kits. Anesth Analg 2012;114:1073–80.
[29] Sustainable Development Unit. Greenhouse gas accounting sector guidance for pharmaceutical products and medical devices. London (England): National Health Service; 2012.
[30] Sulbaek Andersen MP, Nielsen OJ, Karpichev B, et al. Atmospheric chemistry of isoflurane, desflurane, and sevoflurane: kinetics and mechanisms of reactions with chlorine atoms and OH radicals and global warming potentials. J Phys Chem A 2012;116:5806–20.
[31] Ryan SM, Nielsen CJ. Global warming potential of inhaled anesthetics: application to clinical use. Anesth Analg 2010;111:92–8.
[32] Sherman J, Eckelman M. Estimate of carbon dioxide equivalents of inhaled anesthetics in the United States. San Francisco (CA): American Society of Anesthesiologists; 2014.
[33] Sulbaek Andersen MP, Sander SP, Nielsen OJ, et al. Inhalation anaesthetics and climate change. Br J Anaesth 2010;105:760–6.
[34] Sulbaek Andersen MP, Nielsen OJ, Wallington TJ, et al. Medical intelligence article: assessing the impact on global climate from general anesthetic gases. Anesth Analg 2012;114:1081–5.
[35] Vollmer MK, Rhee TS, Rigby M, et al. Modern inhalation anesthetics: potent greenhouse gases in the global atmosphere. Geophys Res Lett 2015;42:1606–11.
[36] Ravishankara AR, Daniel JS, Portmann RW. Nitrous Oxide (N2O): the dominant ozone-depleting substance emitted in the 21st century. Science 2009;326:123–5.
[37] Feldman JM. Managing fresh gas flow to reduce environmental contamination. Anesth Analg 2012;114:1093–101.
[38] Ryan S, Sherman J. Sustainable anesthesia. Anesth Analg 2012;114:921–3.
[39] Barwise JA, Lancaster LJ, Michaels D, et al. Technical communication: an initial evaluation of a novel anesthetic scavenging interface. Anesth Analg 2011;113:1064–7.
[40] Deltasorb. Anesthetic Collection Service. Available at: http://bluezone.ca/. Accessed March 28, 2016.
[41] Drugs Therapeutic Committee and the Health and Medical Care Administration of the Stockholm County Council Sweden. Janusinfo. Available at: http://www.janusinfo.se/In-English/. Accessed March 28, 2016.
[42] Bach PB, Conti RM, Muller RJ, et al. Overspending driven by oversized single dose vials of cancer drugs. BMJ 2016;352:i788.
[43] Harris G. Waste in cancer drugs costs $3 billion a year, a study says. New York: New York Times; 2016.
[44] Shen Rastogi N. Do hospitals make too much trash? Available at: http://www.washingtonpost.com/wp-dyn/content/article/2010/10/18/AR2010101805739.html. Accessed March 28, 2016.

[45] US Environmental Protection Agency Section 6604(b)(5) of the PPA USCb: Memorandum of Understanding Between the United States Environmental Protection Agency and the American Hospital Association. 1998.
[46] Sherman J, Raibley L, Eckelman M, et al. Reusable versus disposable laryngoscopes: environmental and economic considerations. Proceedings of the American Society of Anesthesiologists. New Orleans (LA): American Society of Anesthesiologists; 2014.
[47] McGain F, McAlister S, McGavin A, et al. The financial and environmental costs of reusable and single-use plastic anaesthetic drug trays. Anaesth Intensive Care 2010;38:538–44.
[48] US Food and Drug Administration (FDA). FDA-cleared Sterilants and High Level Disinfectants with General Claims for Processing Reusable Medical and Dental Devices, 2009.
[49] General Accounting Office (GOA). Report to the Committee on Oversight and Government Reform, House of Representatives. Reprocessed Single-Use Medical Devices: FDA Oversight Has Increased, and Available Information Does Not Indicate That Use Presents an Elevated Health Risk. Washington, DC: Government Accountability Office; 2008.
[50] Kwakye G, Pronovost PJ, Makary MA. Commentary: a call to go green in health care by reprocessing medical equipment. Acad Med 2010;85:398–400.
[51] Environmental Working Group. Greening hospitals: An analysis of pollution prevention in America's top hospitals. Available at: http://www.ewg.org/research/greening-hospitals. Accessed March 28, 2016.
[52] GGHH. Green Guide for Health Care. Available at: http://www.gghc.org/resources.overview.php. Accessed March 28, 2016.
[53] Husum B, Stenqvist O, Alahuhta S, et al. Current use of nitrous oxide in public hospitals in Scandinavian countries. Acta Anaesthesiol Scand 2013;57:1131–7.
[54] Conzen PF, Kharasch ED, Czerner SF, et al. Low-flow sevoflurane compared with low-flow isoflurane anesthesia in patients with stable renal insufficiency. Anesthesiology 2002;97: 578–84.
[55] Egger Halbeis CB, Macario A, Brock-Utne JG. The reuse of anesthesia breathing systems: another difference of opinion and practice between the United States and Europe. J Clin Anesth 2008;20:81–3.
[56] McGain F, Algie CM, O'Toole J, et al. The microbiological and sustainability effects of washing anaesthesia breathing circuits less frequently. Anaesthesia 2014;69:337–42.
[57] US Green Buildings Council. Leadership in Energy and Environmental Design (LEED). Available at: www.usgbc.org. Accessed March 28, 2016.
[58] Ard JL Jr, Tobin K, Huncke T, et al. A survey of the American Society of Anesthesiologists regarding environmental attitudes, knowledge, and organization. A A Case Rep 2016;6:208–16.
[59] Sherman J. The perioperative garden of eden: leading edge or trailing edge? A A Case Rep 2016;6(7):183–5.

Advances in Anesthesia 34 (2016) 63–83

ADVANCES IN ANESTHESIA

Point-of-Care Ultrasonography in Pediatrics

Amod Sawardekar, MD[a,*], Adam Spencer, MD, MSc, FRCPC[b], Narasimhan Jagannathan, MD[a], Suresh Santhanam, MD[a]

[a]Department of Pediatric Anesthesiology, Ann & Robert H. Lurie Children's Hospital of Chicago, Feinberg School of Medicine, Northwestern University, 225 East Chicago Avenue, Chicago, IL 60611, USA; [b]Alberta Children's Hospital, University of Calgary, 2888 Shaganappi Trail Northwest, Calgary, Alberta T3B 6A8, Canada

Keywords

• Point of care • Pediatric ultrasonography • Pediatric airway management • Antral imaging • Regional anesthesia • Gastric volume measurement • Aspiration

Key points

- Point-of-care ultrasonography can be used for various clinical applications in pediatric anesthesia.
- This article describes how ultrasonography is used in children for gastric imaging, peripheral regional anesthesia, and airway management.
- Antral sonography at the bedside allows for real-time assessment of gastric contents and potential risk for pulmonary aspiration.
- Point-of-care ultrasonography can also be used for established techniques of pediatric regional anesthesia.
- Lastly, sonographic imaging of the pediatric airway can determine airway management in many situations.

INTRODUCTION

The use of ultrasonography has enhanced the clinical practice of pediatric anesthesia. It is most commonly used in performing peripheral regional anesthetics and for obtaining vascular access. Advances in point-of-care (POC) ultrasonography allow pediatric anesthesiologists to complete physiologic and anatomic studies, in addition to these traditional tasks, without patient

*Corresponding author. Department of Pediatric Anesthesiology, Ann & Robert H. Lurie Children's Hospital of Chicago, Feinberg School of Medicine, Northwestern University, 225 East Chicago Avenue, Box 19, Chicago, IL 60611. *E-mail address*: asawardekar@luriechildrens.org

http://dx.doi.org/10.1016/j.aan.2016.07.005
0737-6146/16/

or practitioner exposure to radiation. After understanding the limitations of POC sonography, the clinician can use this tool to provide real-time physiologic information. This review describes its use in antral imaging to determine gastric volumes. This information can then be used to make immediate clinical decisions. Other uses of POC ultrasonography include basic anatomic visualization that is used for peripheral regional anesthesia and for determining airway anatomy for further intervention. The broad knowledge that can be obtained from POC ultrasonography makes it a valuable tool to the everyday practice of anesthesiology.

POINT-OF-CARE ULTRASONOGRAPHY FOR GASTRIC IMAGING

Pediatric patients presenting for emergency procedures requiring sedation or general anesthesia are at risk of pulmonary aspiration [1]. When it does occur, pulmonary aspiration can be associated with significant morbidity and mortality [2,3].

An at-risk stomach, defined as increased gastric volume or the presence of solid or thick liquid gastric content, can increase the risk of aspiration-related complications [4,5]. The upper limit of normal gastric fasting volume is controversial, but data suggest that up to about 1.5 mL/kg in the adult patient [6] and 1.2 mL/kg in the pediatric patient population are considered normal [7,8]. To this end, most institutions have fasting guidelines to reduce the likelihood of patients presenting with an at-risk stomach. Nevertheless, acute care specialists are faced with nebulous situations in which a patient may be at increased risk of aspiration including trauma patients presenting for surgery, patients who are in pain or are receiving opioids, patients with medical conditions such as diabetes that may delay gastric emptying, and situations in which the fasting period is unclear. In these circumstances, antral sonography may present itself as a clinically useful bedside tool to assess a patient's aspiration risk and to help guide airway or anesthetic management [9].

Previously studied methods to determine gastric content or volumes include polyethylene glycol dilution [10], scintigraphic tracing of gastric contents [11], endoscopic and blind aspiration of gastric contents [12], and MRI [13,14]. Compared with other imaging modalities, ultrasonography is readily available, highly accessible, and economical and does not expose the subject to ionizing radiation. In addition, there is a movement toward increased integration of perioperative sonography in various acute care settings with the goal to improve patient care and outcomes. For these reasons, ultrasonography has become a valuable instrument used in the assessment of aspiration risk in adults and special populations such as obstetric, obese, and pediatric patients [6,15].

Antral sonography: sonoanatomy and technique

Antral sonography can be described as a dynamic ultrasound scan in which the goal is to examine the antrum at rest between peristaltic contractions. The antrum can be identified by its 5 sonographic layers that are specific to the stomach [16]. When empty, the 2 outer layers, consisting of the serosa and muscularis propria, are distinct (Fig. 1). The serosa is the outermost layer and presents as a hyperechoic (bright) layer. It is followed by a thick hypoechoic (dark) layer known as the muscularis propria, which is responsible for forceful peristaltic actions. Three additional internal layers can be identified, including the submucosa, muscularis mucosa, and the innermost thin hyperechoic layer highlighting the mucosal–air interface.

The antrum is reliably identified in most patients, including pediatric patients of various ages [14,15,17]. Moreover, the antrum best reflects total gastric volume when compared with the gastric body or fundus [18,19]. Traditionally, the use of a low-frequency curvilinear transducer is often recommended to assess the gastric antrum. However, a recent study of pediatric patients over a wide age range suggests that a better view of the antrum is achieved with a high-frequency linear transducer (high frequency, 7–12 MHz) in younger patients ($\bar{X}$ 8.5 years; 95% confidence interval [CI], 7.1–9.9 years), likely caused by the more superficial position of the antrum [20]. A better view was gained with a curvilinear transducer (low frequency, 2–5 MHz) in older children ($\bar{X}$ 13.1 years; 95% CI, 11.7–14.6 years).

The scan should be completed with the patient in the supine and in the right lateral decubitus (RLD) positions (Fig. 2). With the transducer positioned in a para-sagittal scanning plane in the epigastric region, the antrum can be found between the left lobe of the liver and the pancreas at the level of the aorta or the inferior vena cava (IVC). Visualization of vascular landmarks including

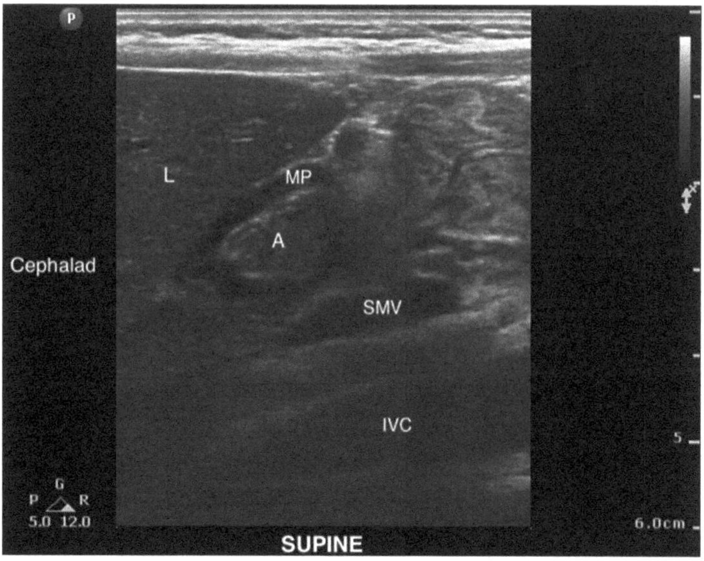

Fig. 1. Ultrasound image of the empty antrum with patient in the supine position. A, antrum; IVC, inferior vena cava; L, liver; MP, muscularis propria; SMV, superior mesenteric vein.

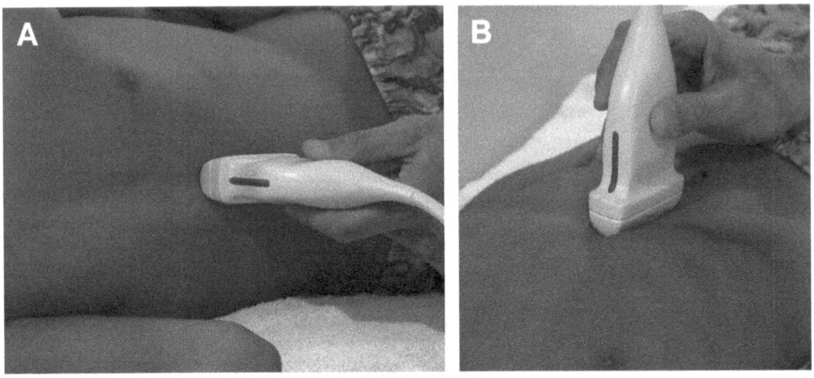

Fig. 2. (*A*) Probe position with patient in the right lateral decubitus position. (*B*) Probe position with patient in the supine position.

the abdominal aorta, IVC, and either the superior mesenteric artery or superior mesenteric vein has been used to standardize a scanning plane through the antrum [18]. Compared with the IVC, the wall of the abdominal aorta appears thicker, hyperechoic, and pulsatile and is typically found slightly to the left of the IVC and of the vertebral body. The IVC is also more compressible, its shape changes with respiration, and gentle cephalic tilting of the transducer while following this vessel will image its proximal portion merging into the right atrium. When the antrum is identified, the sonographer should ensure that only gentle pressure is used so as not to compress the antrum, as this can produce false information, especially when measuring its cross-sectional area (CSA) for the purpose of predicting gastric volume.

Basic scanning movements with the transducer

The scanning technique is similar to that described for adults [6]. Initially, the transducer should lie in a parasagittal scanning plane in the right subcostal margin. From this position, slide the transducer from the patient's right subcostal margin toward the patient's abdominal midline and up to the left subcostal margin. By convention, the liver should immediately be seen on the left side of the monitor. As the transducer slowly moves across the epigastric area, a search for vascular structures such as the IVC, aorta, and superior mesenteric artery should be completed. The antrum should be seen between the left lobe of the liver and the pancreas and carefully inspected for the presence of contents when at the level of the IVC or abdominal aorta.

Assessment of the antral content

As described in a recent review [6], antral sonography initially involves a qualitative assessment to verify whether the antrum appears empty or contains fluid or solid contents. Although it is customary to perform a physical examination on patients in the supine position, it is important not to rely on findings of antral sonography based on this position without assessing the patient in the RLD position [6]. A significant amount of content (both fluid and solid) may be present in the fundus and may only become apparent in the antrum when the patient is turned to the RLD position [5,15].

Empty = low-risk situation
An empty antrum appears flat with abutting anterior and posterior walls and is described as a *bull's eye* shape (see Fig. 1) [21]. The muscularis propria also appears thicker when the antrum is empty. This finding in both the supine and RLD positions suggests a low-risk situation for pulmonary aspiration in which measurement of the antral CSA is not required.

Thick fluid or solid = high-risk situation
Thick fluid or solid contents have a high or mixed echogenicity. If the stomach contains a thicker type of fluid such as milk, this liquid content may appear slightly hyperechoic. A frosted-glass appearance caused by air artifact may suggest an at-risk stomach and can be caused by a mixture of air and solid contents, which is typical after the ingestion of solid or thicker liquids [18]. This air artifact makes it difficult to assess the posterior wall and very challenging to perform a measurement of the antral CSA used to predict total gastric volume. The presence of thick fluid or solid contents suggests an at-risk stomach with an increased risk of aspiration, regardless of the total volume of gastric contents.

Clear fluid = equivocal risk
When clear fluid is present, the antrum appears distended with anechoic fluid (Fig. 3). Typically, as the patient moves from the supine to the RLD position, the antrum appears larger as the fluid shifts toward the more dependent antrum region of the stomach. In this case, a quantitative volume assessment may help distinguish a low volume, consistent with the volume of gastric secretions in the supine position, or a higher-than-baseline volume in the RLD position, which could increase a patient's aspiration risk.

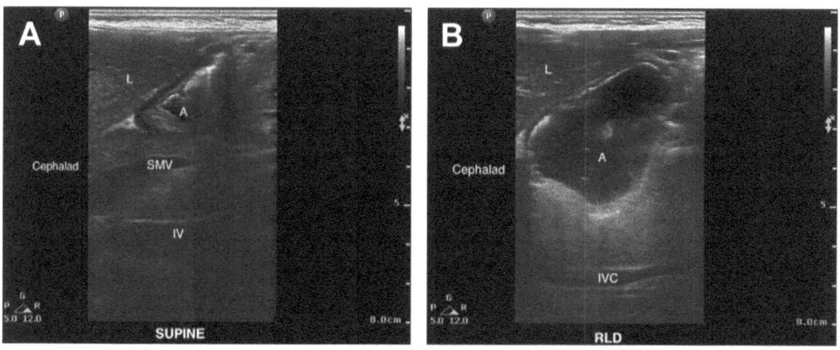

Fig. 3. (*A*) Gastric image with the patient in the supine position. (*B*) Gastric image with the patient in the lateral decubitus position. A, antrum; IVC, inferior vena cava; L, liver; MP, muscularis propria; SMV, superior mesenteric vein.

Predicting gastric volume based on antral cross-sectional area

Antral CSA should be measured while in a relaxed state between peristaltic contractions. Two methods are described including (1) measuring 2 perpendicular diameters using both the anterior-posterior and cranio-caudal planes from serosa to serosa and (2) using a free trace tool and outlining the serosal border of the antrum to produce a CSA [6].

Several studies in various adult and pediatric populations investigated the correlation between antral CSA and total gastric volume [6]. Three pediatric studies [14,15,22] found correlation coefficients ranging from 0.67 to 0.91. Similar to adult studies, correlation coefficients were strongest when patients were examined while in the RLD position [6]. Two of the studies produced mathematical models using antral CSA in RLD position to predict gastric volume [14,15]. Spencer and colleagues [15] examined the relationship between sonographically measured antral CSA and gastric fluid volume suctioned under endoscopic guidance. Multiple regression analysis was used to develop a mathematical model that estimates gastric volume based on antral CSA in RLD position and patient's age ($R^2 = 0.60$).

$$\text{Volume} = -7.8 + (3.5 \text{ x RLD CSA}) + (0.127) \text{ x age (months)}$$

Although promising, this is a preliminary model that should be further validated in nonfasting pediatric patients with increased gastric volumes before using results to guide clinical decision making in emergent situations [15].

Estimating total gastric volume (milliliters per kilogram) based on antral CSA would be ideal; however, because of limited pediatric data, a qualitative assessment may be more clinically useful at this time. A recent review of antral sonography [6] proposed a semiquantitative algorithm for the application of this POC tool using a 3-point grading system. This grading system was assessed previously in adults [5,7] and was also found to correlate with gastric volumes in children [15]. The system is based on the appearance of antral content in both supine and RLD positions. A grading of 0, 1, or 2 is applied as follows: grade 0: no fluid visible in the antrum in either the supine or RLD position, which indicates a low gastric volume state. Grade 1: antral fluid visualized only in the RLD position may represent a normal gastric volume but a quantitative volume assessment may help differentiate a normal from a high gastric volume in this setting. Grade 2: antral fluid visualized in both the supine and RLD positions assumes a higher gastric volume. Mean gastric volumes (milliliters per kilogram, interquartile range) differed significantly between the 3 groups in the pediatric study: grade 0: $\overline{X} = 0.3$ mL/kg (0.2), grade 1: $\overline{X} = 0.7$ mL/kg (0.4), and grade 2: $\overline{X} = 1.5$ mL/kg (1.4) [15]. Although additional studies are needed, these results suggest that this grading system can be a useful bedside tool to differentiate a low (grade 0) from a high (grade 2) gastric volume setting [5].

Antral sonography completed at a patient's bedside is a readily available and noninvasive tool that can be used to assess gastric content and volume and to provide an aspiration risk assessment when this would add to the quality of the historical and clinical information. Although additional pediatric studies are needed to further validate gastric sonography in children presenting with potentially full stomachs, antral sonography can be effectively used to determine both gastric content (empty, fluid, solid) and whether the patient may have a larger than normal gastric volume to help guide anesthetic or airway management.

POINT-OF-CARE ULTRASONOGRAPHY FOR REGIONAL ANESTHESIA

POC ultrasonography has contributed to the increasing utilization of regional anesthesia techniques in pediatric patients. The introduction of ultrasonography increases the applicability for performing peripheral nerve blockade in children. Use of the ultrasound scan facilitates real-time navigation of a needle to the desired neural structure. This technique is of particular value in pediatric anesthesia to support regional anesthesia techniques, as it is so common that these procedures are completed while children are anesthetized [23,24].

Although literature evaluating the evidence for success and safety of ultrasonography in regional anesthesia is emerging through various sources, the pediatric regional anesthesia network has collected data demonstrating safety and efficacy of many regional anesthesia techniques [25]. In addition to case series and clinical studies, descriptions from case reports may increase awareness of areas in which ultrasonography may be used in performing regional anesthesia in children.

UPPER EXTREMITY PERIPHERAL BLOCKADE

Axillary block

Nerve blockade at the axillary location of the brachial plexus allows for analgesia to the elbow, forearm, and hand. A single needle insertion permits blockade of the radial, median, and ulnar nerves; however, the musculocutaneous nerve is usually spared. Once the axillary artery is identified, the radial nerve can be found posterior to it, and the ulnar nerve is anterior and inferior. The median nerve is found anterior and superior to the axillary artery. The musculocutaneous nerve is found between the biceps brachii and coracobrachialis muscles and often requires a separate needle insertion to be blocked.

Ultrasound-guided axillary blocks in children follow techniques described for adults, as there are limited descriptions for pediatric patients [26,27]. An out-of-plane technique is used with the ultrasound probe placed transverse to the humerus. A single needle insertion with multiple injections allows for spread of local anesthetic within the neurovascular sheath [6]. The needle can be advanced with direct visualization when ultrasonography is used (Fig. 4).

Complications include hematoma, infection at the site of skin puncture, skin tenderness, neural injury, and intravascular injection. The use of ultrasound guidance for real-time visualization may decrease the risk of intravascular injection and nerve damage.

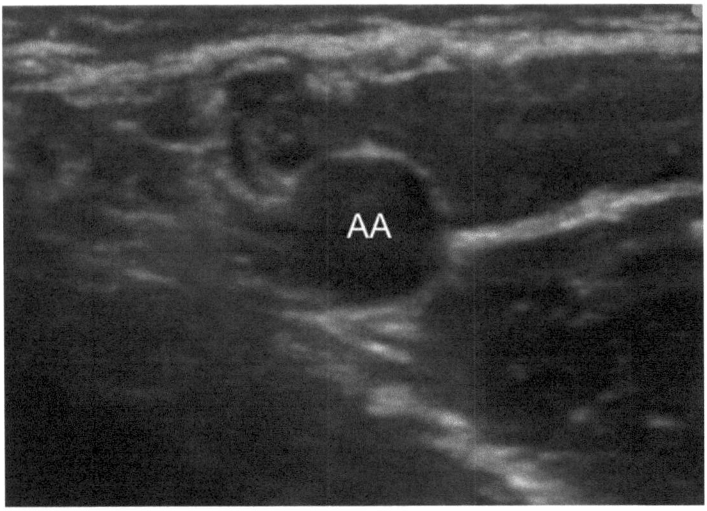

Fig. 4. Ultrasound image of the brachial plexus in the axilla. AA, axillary artery.

Interscalene approach

The interscalene block is frequently used to provide analgesia to the shoulder and upper arm by blocking the roots and trunks of the brachial plexus. In this location, the brachial plexus is positioned deep to the sternocleidomastoid muscle between the anterior and middle scalene muscles.

The ultrasound probe is placed at the lateral aspect of the sternocleidomastoid muscle at the level of the cricoid cartilage in the transverse oblique plane. The anterior and medial scalene muscles are then identified deep to these structures, which make up the borders of the interscalene groove (Fig. 5). Within the groove are the C5, C6, and C7 nerve roots of the brachial plexus. An in-plane or out-of-plane approach can be used to advance the needle to the brachial plexus in this location. In addition, the use of ultrasonography may allow for a reduced local anesthetic requirement to achieve satisfactory block [28].

Successful blockade is accompanied by hemidiaphragmatic paralysis, recurrent laryngeal nerve block, and Horner syndrome [29]. In addition to the risks of vascular puncture and infection, the interscalene block should be used with caution because of the potential risks of pneumothorax, vertebral artery injection, and intrathecal injection.

Supraclavicular approach

The supraclavicular approach is the most common approach to the brachial plexus in children and provides analgesia to the upper arm and elbow. The common visualized landmark is the subclavian artery and just lateral and superficial to it are the trunks and divisions of the plexus (Fig. 6). The first rib and pleura are seen deep to the plexus and the subclavian artery.

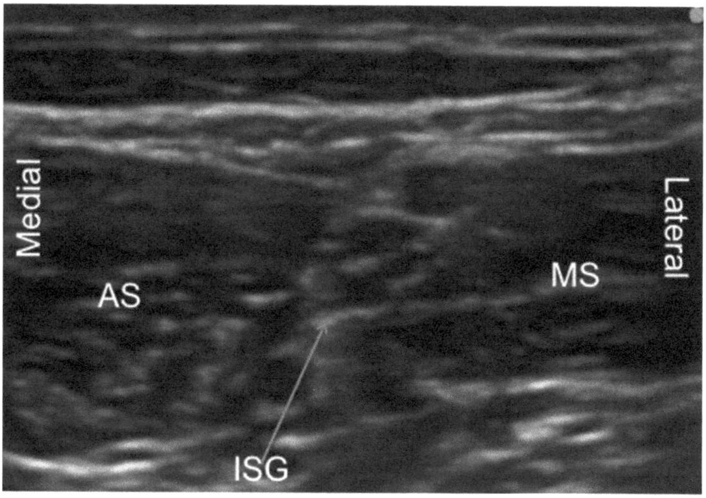

Fig. 5. Ultrasound image of the brachial plexus from the interscalene approach. AS, anterior scalene muscle; ISG, interscalene groove; MS, middle scalene muscle.

Few techniques are described in the pediatric population [30]. The ultrasound probe is placed superior to the midclavicle in the coronal oblique plane. The subclavian artery is identified as the hypoechoic pulsatile structure. A needle can be advanced from a lateral position and directed medially using

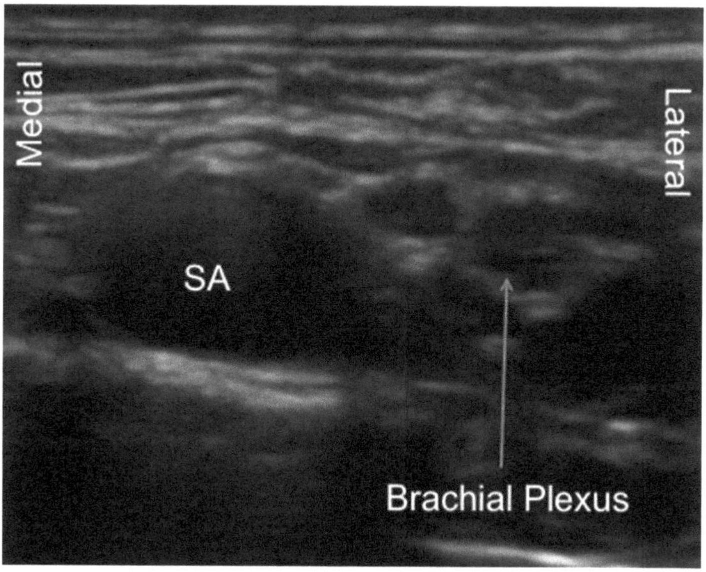

Fig. 6. Ultrasound image of the brachial plexus in the supraclavicular fossa. SA, subclavian artery.

an in-plane approach toward the brachial plexus. This technique lowers the risk of vascular and intraneural injection.

Complications include hematoma, infection, and intravascular injection. In addition, completion of the supraclavicular block confers an increased risk of pneumothorax, as the lung parenchyma lies just medial to the first rib at the level at which the block is completed [31,32]. For this reason, visualization of the tip and shaft of the needle with ultrasonography may aid in its prevention.

Infraclavicular approach

Just inferior to the coracoid process, the brachial plexus cords can be found. The axillary artery and vein surround the cords of the brachial plexus. Superficial to these structures are the pectoralis major and minor. The lateral cord of the plexus is seen on the ultrasound scan as a hyperechoic structure, and the posterior cord is positioned deep to the axillary artery. The medial cord is located between the axillary artery and vein, which can make it difficult to identify with ultrasonography. An infraclavicular approach is often preferred for indwelling catheter placement, as a catheter in this location is less prone to displacement with neck movement.

Multiple techniques have been described for an infraclavicular approach to the brachial plexus. Depending on the expertise and familiarity of the clinician, an in-plane or out-of-plane approach can be used [30,33]. With either technique, care should be taken to avoid vascular structures and the pleura.

Similar to the supraclavicular block, complications include hematoma, infection, and intravascular injection. The risk of a pneumothorax persists because of the proximity of the cervical pleura.

Transversus abdominis plane block

The transversus abdominis plane block provides analgesia to the anterior abdominal wall and is commonly used as pain relief for abdominal incisions, including laparoscopic port placement [34,35]. Lateral to rectus abdominis muscles lie 3 muscle layers: the external oblique, internal oblique, and tranversus abdominis. The thoracolumbar nerve roots (T8–L1) course through the internal oblique and transversus abdominis muscle layers (Fig. 7).

Often, an in-plane approach with ultrasound guidance is used to guide needle advancement to the transverse abdominis plane [34,36]. A linear, high-frequency probe is placed lateral to the rectus abdominis to identify the peritoneal cavity, and superficial to this are the 3 muscle layers. Injection, with incremental aspiration, will create an elliptical pocket of local anesthetic in the compartment that the nerves traverse. Ultrasonography with direct visualization may limit the incidence of complications such as intravascular injection and peritoneal or bowel puncture [34,37].

Ilioinguinal/iliohypogastric nerve block

The ilioinguinal/iliohypogastric (IL/IH) nerves originate from T12 and L1 and course the internal oblique aponeurosis at the level of the anterior superior iliac spine (ASIS). IL/IH nerve blocks provide analgesia for surgical procedures in

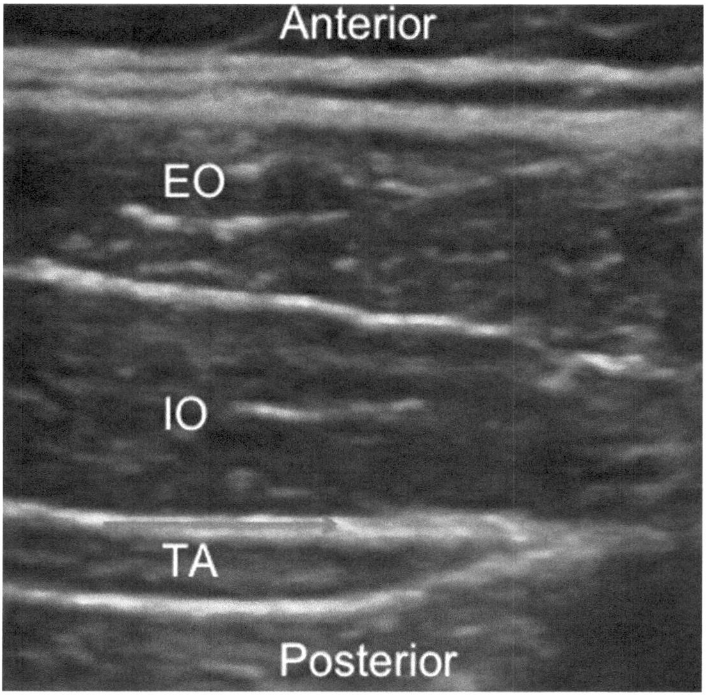

Fig. 7. Ultrasound image of the anterior abdominal wall. EO, external oblique muscle; IO, internal oblique muscle; TA, transversus abdominus muscle. (*Arrow* pointing to the transverse abdominis plane.)

the inguinal region and anterior scrotum. A linear ultrasound probe is placed at the level of the ASIS in line with the umbilicus. Medial to the ASIS shadow, the inguinal nerve may appear as an ovular structure between the internal oblique and transverse abdominal muscles (Fig. 8). The needle is inserted using an in-plane technique and advanced to the nerve. The volume of local anesthetic solution used to anesthetize both nerves is significantly reduced with the use of ultrasonography [38,39]. Use of ultrasonography can reduce effective volume of local anesthetic to as low as 0.075 mL/kg [40,41]. Rare complications include pelvic hematoma and femoral nerve palsy.

Rectus sheath block

The rectus sheath block provides analgesia for midline abdominal procedures. It is commonly used for periumbilical surgical procedures including single-incision laparoscopic surgery and umbilical hernia repair [42]. The rectus abdominis muscle is separated in the midline by the linea alba, and the thoracolumbar nerves (T7-T11) travel the potential space between the rectus abdominis muscle and posterior sheath. A high-frequency linear probe is placed lateral to the umbilicus, and the rectus abdominis muscle is seen as the first major layer beyond the subcutaneous tissue. The posterior sheath lies just below

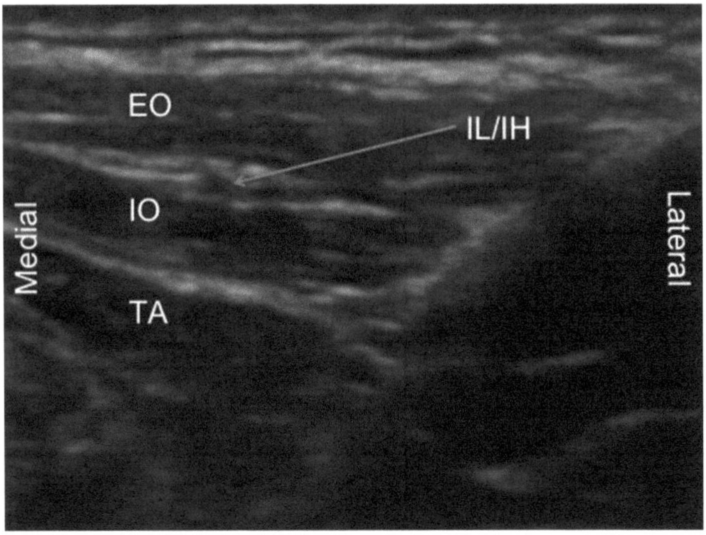

Fig. 8. Ultrasound image of the IL/IH nerve block. EO, external oblique muscle; IO, internal oblique muscle; TA, transversus abdominus muscle.

the rectus abdominis and above the peritoneum (Fig. 9). A needle is advanced using an in-plane technique, and local anesthetic is deposited in the potential space between the rectus abdominis muscle and its posterior sheath. Approximately 0.1 mL/kg of local anesthetic is used to provide analgesia [43]. Complications include bowel puncture and intravascular injection caused by the proximity of the inferior epigastric artery.

Femoral nerve block

The femoral nerve originates from nerve roots L2, L3, and L4, and its block provides analgesia from the anterior thigh to the knee. The femoral nerve is located lateral to the femoral artery and vein. With a linear probe placed in the inguinal crease, the femoral artery is identified as the pulsatile structure, and just lateral to the artery is the femoral nerve (Fig. 10) [44]. An in-plane or out-of-plane technique is used to advance a needle and to visualize local anesthetic injection to surround the femoral nerve [45]. Care is taken to identify the large vascular structures around the nerve to avoid vessel puncture and hematoma formation.

Saphenous nerve block

The saphenous nerve provides innervation to the knee, the medial portion of the leg below the knee, and the medial portion of the foot. It is a sensory branch of the femoral nerve and travels within the adductor canal, running next to the sartorius muscle before continuing to the medial aspect of the knee. Using ultrasonography, the nerve can be identified in the proximal thigh to provide

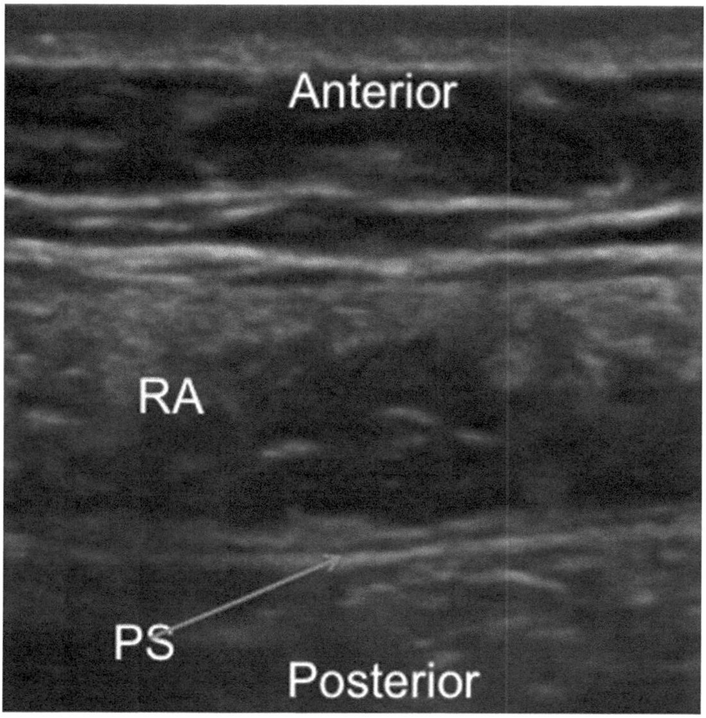

Fig. 9. Ultrasound image of the anterior abdominal wall. PS, posterior sheath; RA, rectus abdominus muscle.

sensory analgesia to the anterior knee, or it can be identified distally to provide analgesia to the medial aspect of the lower extremity [46]. The patient is placed in the supine position with the leg abducted and laterally rotated, and the probe is placed on the medial aspect of the knee. The saphenous nerve is identified posterior to the sartorius muscle, and the needle is directed to the saphenous nerve using an in-plane technique, where local anesthetic is deposited. Complications include nerve injury, hematoma from arterial puncture, and infection.

Sciatic nerve blocks

The sciatic nerve originates from the nerve roots of L4 to S3, and when blocked provides analgesia to the posterior thigh and all but the medial aspect of the leg distal to the knee. The sciatic nerve exits the pelvis in the greater sciatic foramen and courses inferior to the gluteus maximus muscle. The sciatic nerve bifurcates, proximal to the popliteal fossa, into the tibial and common peroneal nerves (Fig. 11). The sciatic nerve can be blocked at the subgluteal or popliteal locations in children but is often more superficial in the popliteal fossa, allowing for better visualization with POC ultrasonography [47]. This visualization is accomplished with the patient in the supine or prone

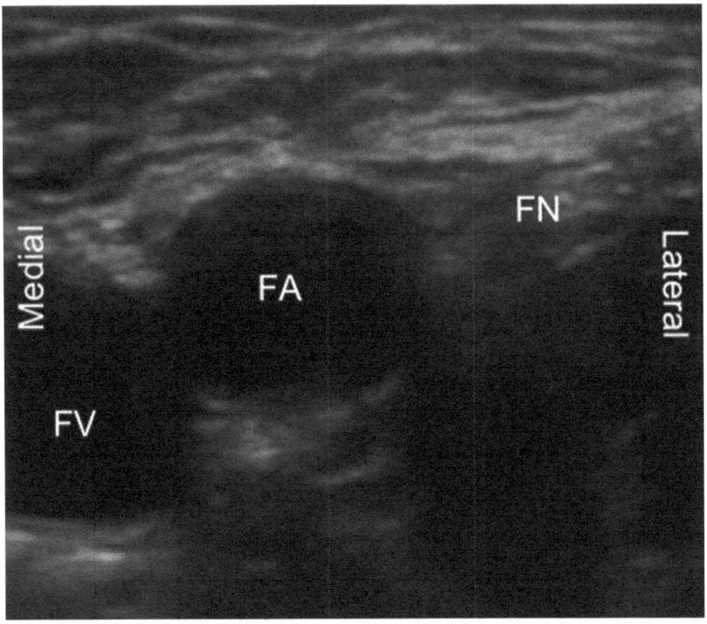

Fig. 10. Ultrasound image of the femoral nerve. FA, femoral artery; FN, femoral nerve; FV, femoral vein.

position with the ultrasound probe placed above the popliteal crease. The popliteal artery is identified as the pulsatile structure and then the tibial nerve is visualized next to the artery. Imaging more proximally, the tibial and common peroneal nerves are seen joining to form the sciatic nerve [48,49]. An in-plane technique can be used to guide the needle under direct visualization and to image local anesthetic injection to surround the nerves. Complications from any of these approaches include infection, hematoma from vessel puncture, and local anesthetic toxicity.

POINT-OF-CARE ULTRASONOGRAPHY FOR AIRWAY MANAGEMENT

Ultrasonography is a portable and reliable modality to allow imaging of the larynx, vocal cords, and trachea and the assessment of dynamic changes at the bedside. Visualization of the changes of anatomy and locations in real time is a distinct advantage when using ultrasonography. However, 2 operators are often needed: one to handle to probe and the other to instrument the airway, which can be impractical during airway management. Pediatric anesthesiologists, emergency medicine physicians, pediatric intensive care physicians, and paramedics may all benefit from use of airway ultrasonography use in children.

This brief review describes scanning of the larynx and subglottic region, with a discussion of the potential clinical applications of airway ultrasonography.

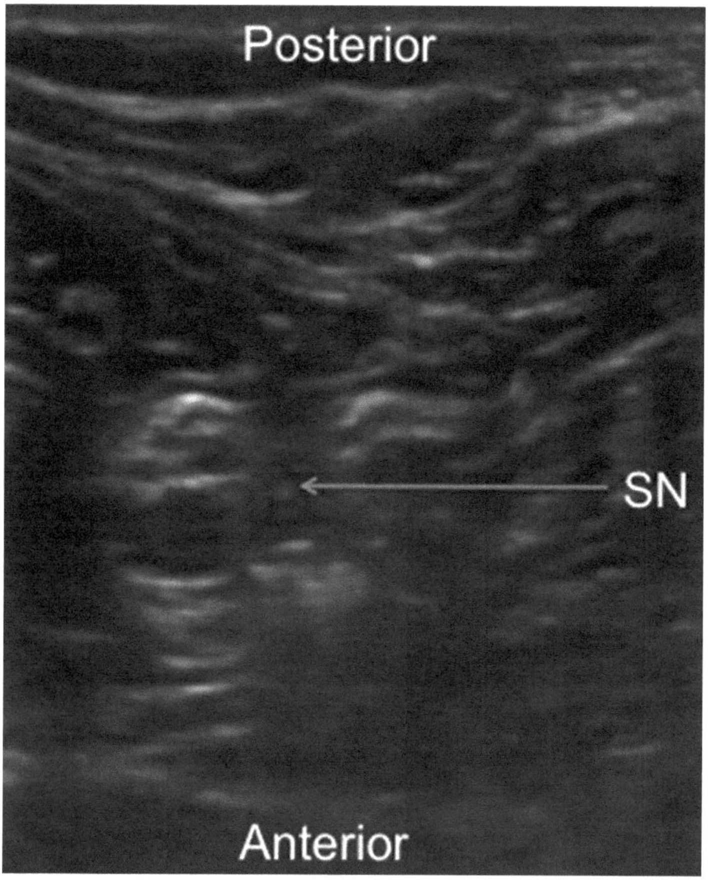

Fig. 11. Ultrasound image of the sciatic nerve (SN).

Basic considerations

A. Position

Patients should be placed in supine sniffing position to achieve slight head extension.

B. Equipment

Two types of probes commonly used are linear and curved. A standard 7.5-MHz linear probe and a 5-MHz curved probe are commonly used for visualization of superficial and deeper structures of the airway, respectively. A planar linear high-frequency (4–15 MHz) transducer allows for good resolution and image detail of superficial structures and is the most versatile probe for showing airway structures in children.

C. Transducer orientation

Sagittal view (longitudinally in the midline) and transverse view (transversely across the anterior surface of the neck) are used.

Areas to scan

Infrahyoid region

In the transverse view, the hyoid bone appears hypoechoic, as it is still relatively cartilaginous in small children. As it calcifies, it increases in echogenicity and casts a posterior acoustic shadow. Beneath the hyoid, images can be obtained in transverse and longitudinal plains allowing for visualization of the larynx and its internal structures.

A transverse view also allows identification of the upper larynx, false vocal cords superiorly, true vocal cords inferiorly, and the upper trachea and esophagus at the level of the thyroid gland. The true cords (Fig. 12) are inferior to the false cords. The arytenoid cartilages can also be appreciated in this region.

Trachea

In the transverse view, the trachea comes into sight as the probe is oriented inferiorly from the lower larynx. The thyroid gland surrounding the trachea is easily identified. The hypoechoic (dark) anterior part of each tracheal ring can be easily identified, but the tracheal walls are not as well demarcated, secondary to air seen centrally. The esophagus can be identified as being left and posteromedial to the trachea (multilayered structure). The carotid arteries are seen posterolateral to the thyroid lobes (Fig. 13).

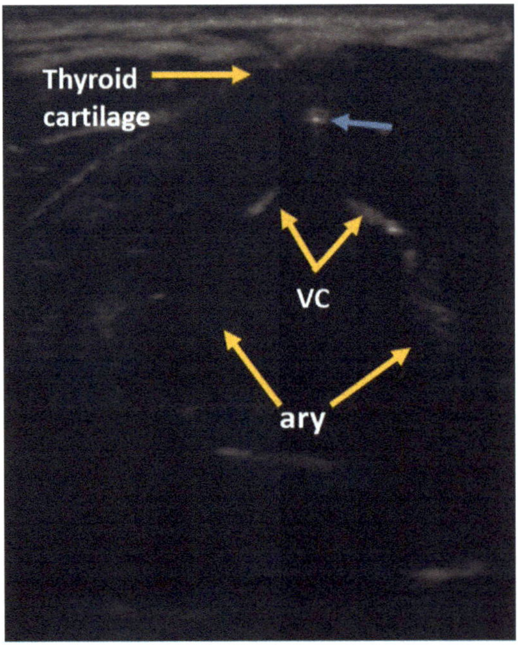

Fig. 12. Transverse view of the upper larynx: vocal cords and arytenoid cartilages. The thyroid cartilage appears echogenic. The true cords (VC) appear hyperechoic. The area of echogenicity at the superior margin represents the anterior commissure of the vocal cords (*blue arrow*). The areas of echogenicity lateral to the vocal cords represent the arytenoid cartilages (ary).

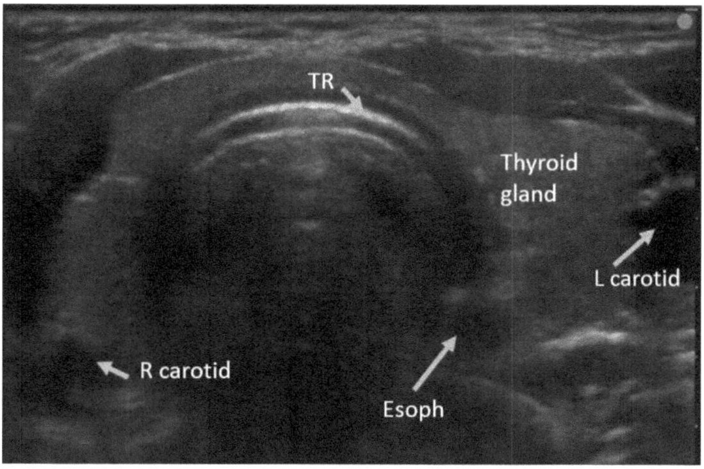

Fig. 13. Transverse view of the lower larynx: trachea, esophagus, and thyroid gland. The echogenic tracheal rings (TR) are easily seen. The esophagus (Esoph) is seen posteromedial and to the left of the trachea. The carotid arteries are seen posterolateral to the thyroid gland lobes.

In the midline longitudinal view, the larynx and upper trachea can be appreciated in the following order from cranial to caudal: thyroid cartilage, cricothyroid membrane, and cricoid cartilage tracheal rings. Between the cricoid cartilage and the thyroid cartilage, the thin cricothyroid membrane can be identified. Just deep to these structures is a continuous bright line from air within the airways (Fig. 14).

Clinical applications of airway ultrasonography in children

Selection of the optimal diameter of tracheal tubes

Because the internal diameter of the trachea can reliably be determined using ultrasonography, identification of subglottic narrowing is possible. It should be emphasized that this application seems to be more useful when uncuffed endotracheal tubes are being used (less useful for cuffed endotracheal tubes). Pediatric patients with tracheostomies may benefit from this ultrasound examination when up- or down-sizing tracheostomy tubes [50,51].

Detection of tracheal intubation/esophageal intubation

Ultrasonography has been described to verify and observe tracheal and inadvertent esophageal intubation [52,53]. Real-time scanning allows visualization of passage of the endotracheal tube between the vocal cords, as evidenced by a change in glottic width. An esophageal intubation may be detected by visualization of the tube in the paratracheal space. Additionally, the use of ultrasonography to verify tracheal intubation may be superior to auscultation in a noisy environment (eg, prehospital helicopter) or in low perfusion states when capnography may be unreliable [54].

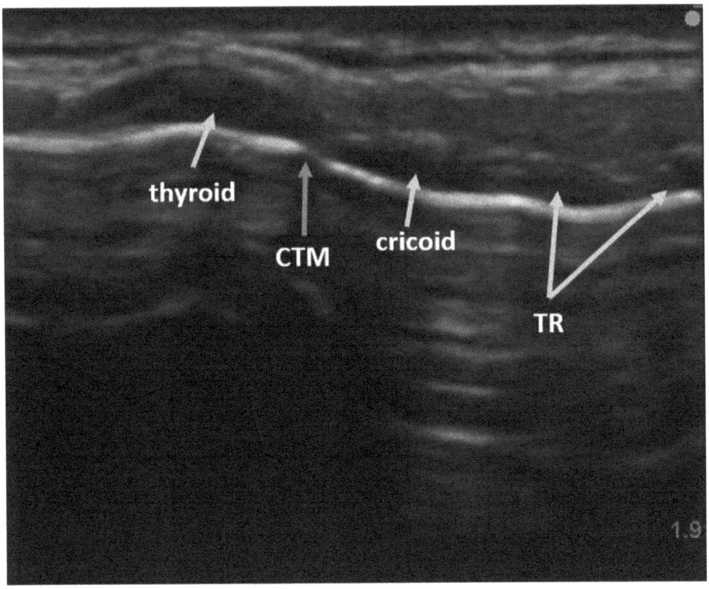

Fig. 14. Midline longitudinal view of the trachea: from (left to right/cranial to caudal): thyroid cartilage (thyroid), cricothyroid membrane (CTM; in between the thyroid and cricoid cartilages), cricoid cartilage (cricoid), and tracheal rings (TR). Just deep to these structures is a continuous bright line from air within the airways.

Tracheal tube depth

The tip of the tracheal tube in relation to the aortic arch, when measured with ultrasonography, can be used to confirm appropriate depth of insertion of the endotracheal tube [55].

Vocal cord movement

Laryngeal ultrasonography can be an adjunct in the assessment of vocal cord paralysis in the pediatric population [56]. It can be used after total thyroidectomy to assess vocal cord movement in the evaluation of recurrent laryngeal nerve function.

Difficult intubation

Ultrasound-guided endotracheal intubation was described in a patient in whom both direct and video laryngoscopy failed. It also may be useful in circumstances in which secretions or blood obscure visualization or if advanced airway equipment (videolaryngoscope/fiberoptic bronchoscope) is unavailable or fails [57].

Supraglottic airway malposition

Ultrasonography has been used to accurately detect when a supraglottic airway device (eg, laryngeal mask airway [LMA]) is rotated out of proper position. This is typically evidenced by ventral movement of the arytenoids resulting in an asymmetric elevation of an arytenoid cartilage [58].

FUTURE APPLICATIONS

Similar to that in the adult population, in children, ultrasonography may aid in the prediction of difficult endotracheal intubation through identification of pre-existing airway lesions or in assessment of the hyomental mobility observed during flexion and extension [59]. Children with known difficult airways may benefit from sonographic identification of the cricothyroid membrane and the location and depth of the trachea if invasive airway access is required during airway management.

References

[1] Warner MA, Warner ME, Warner DO, et al. Perioperative pulmonary aspiration in infants and children. Anesthesiology 1999;90:66–71.

[2] Kozlow J, Berenholtz S, Garrett E, et al. Epidemiology and impact of aspiration pneumonia in patients undergoing surgery in Maryland. Crit Care Med 2003;31:1930–7.

[3] Lienhart A, Auroy Y, Pequignot F, et al. Survey of anesthesia related mortality in France. Anesthesiology 2006;105:1087–97.

[4] Cotton BR, Smith G. The lower oesophageal sphincter and anaesthesia. Br J Anaesth 1984;56:37–46.

[5] Perlas A, Mitsakakis N, Liu L, et al. Validation of a mathematical model for ultrasound assessment of gastric volume by gastroscopic examination. Anesth Analg 2013;116:357–63.

[6] Van de Putte P, Perlas A. Ultrasound assessment of gastric content and volume. Br J Anaesth 2014;113:12–22.

[7] Cook-Sather SD, Liacouras CA, Previte JP, et al. Gastric fluid measurement by blind aspiration: a gastroscopic evaluation. Can J Anaesth 1997;44:168–72.

[8] Schwartz DA, Connelly NR, Theroux CA, et al. Gastric contents in children presenting for upper endoscopy. Anesth Analg 1998;87:757–60.

[9] Alakkad H, Kruisselbrink R, Chin KJ, et al. Point-of-care ultrasound defines gastric content and changes the anesthetic management of elective surgical patients who have not followed fasting instructions: a prospective case series. Can J Anaesth 2015;62:1188–95.

[10] Hardy JF, Plourde G, Lebrun M, et al. Determining gastric contents during general anaesthesia: evaluation of two methods. Can J Anaesth 1987;34:474–7.

[11] Abell TL, Camilleri M, Donohoe K, et al. Consensus recommendations for gastric emptying scintigraphy: a joint report of the American neurogastroenterology and motility society and the society of nuclear medicine. Am J Gastroenterol 2008;103:753–63.

[12] Taylor WJ, Champion MC, Barry AW, et al. Measuring gastric contents during general anaesthesia: evaluation of blind gastric aspiration. Can J Anaesth 1989;36:51–4.

[13] Fidler J, Bharucha AE, Camilleri M, et al. Application of magnetic resonance imaging to measure fasting and postprandial volumes in humans. Neurogastroenterol Motil 2009;21:42–51.

[14] Schmitz A, Thomas S, Melanie F, et al. Ultrasonographic gastric antral area and gastric contents volume in children. Paediatr Anaesth 2012;22:144–9.

[15] Spencer A, Walker AM, Yeung AK, et al. Ultrasound assessment of gastric volume in the fasted pediatric patient undergoing upper gastrointestinal endoscopy: development of a predictive model using endoscopically-suctioned volumes. Paediatr Anaesth 2015;25:301–8.

[16] Cubillos J, Tse C, Chan VW, et al. Bedside ultrasound assessment of gastric content: an observational study. Can J Anaesth 2012;59:416–23.

[17] Arys B, Mandelstam S, Rao P, et al. Sonography of the pediatric gastrointestinal system. Ultrasound Q 2014;30:101–17.

[18] Perlas A, Chan VW, Lupu CM, et al. Ultrasound assessment of gastric content and volume. Anesthesiology 2009;111:82–9.

[19] Sporea I, Popescu A. Ultrasound examination of the normal gastrointestinal tract. Med Ultrason 2010;12:349–52.
[20] Spencer AO, Walker AM. Antral sonography in the pediatric patient: can transducer choice affect the view? Br J Anaesth 2015;114:1002–3.
[21] Ratzlaff RA, Builes A, Diaz-Gomez JL. Current practical applications of ultrasonography in surgical anesthesia. Adv Anesth 2015;33:129–55.
[22] Tomomasa T, Tabata M, Nako Y, et al. Ultrasonographic assessment of intragastric volume in neonates: factors affecting the relationship between intragastric volume and antral cross-sectional area. Pediatr Radiol 1996;26:815–20.
[23] Tsui B, Suresh S. Ultrasound imaging for regional anesthesia in infants, children, and adolescents: a review of current literature and its application to neuraxial blocks. Anesthesiology 2010;112:719–28.
[24] Roberts S. Ultrasonographic guidance in pediatric regional anesthesia. Part 2: techniques. Paediatr Anaesth 2006;16:1112–24.
[25] Polaner DM, Taenzer AH, Walker BJ, et al. Pediatric regional anesthesia network(PRAN): a multi-institutional study of the use and incidence of complications of pediatric regional anesthesia. Anesth Analg 2012;115(6):1353–64.
[26] O'Donnell BD, Iohom G. An estimation of the minimum effective anesthetic volume of 2% lidocaine in ultrasound-guided axillary brachial plexus block. Anesthesiology 2009;111: 25–9.
[27] Van Geffen GJ, Tielens L, Gielen M. Ultrasound-guided interscalene brachial plexus block in a child with femur fibula ulna syndrome. Paediatr Anaesth 2006;16:330–2.
[28] McNaught A, Shastri U, Carmichael N, et al. Ultrasound reduces the minimum effective local anesthetic volume compared with peripheral nerve stimulation for interscalene block. Br J Anaesth 2011;106:124–30.
[29] Fredrickson MJ. Ultrasound-assisted interscalene catheter placement in a child. Anaesth Intensive Care 2007;35:807–8.
[30] De José María B, Banus E, Navarro EM, et al. Ultrasound-guided supraclavicular *vs* infraclavicular brachial plexus blocks in children. Paediatr Anaesth 2008;18:838–44.
[31] Rapp H, Grau T. Ultrasound-guided regional anesthesia in pediatric patients. Tech Reg Anesth Pain Manag 2004;8:179–98.
[32] Marhofer P. Upper extremity peripheral blocks. Tech Reg Anesth Pain Manag 2007;11: 215–21.
[33] Marhofer P, Sitzwohl C, Greher M, et al. Ultrasound guidance for infraclavicular brachial plexus anaethesia in children. Anaesthesia 2004;59:642–6.
[34] Suresh S, Chan VW. Ultrasound guided transversus abdominis plane block in infants, children and adolescents: a simple procedural guidance for their performance. Paediatr Anaesth 2009;19(1):296–9.
[35] Long JB, Schaldenbrand K, Birmingham P, et al. A descriptive analysis of transversus abdominis plane (TAP) blocks in infants, children, and adolescents; lessons learned from the pediatric regional anesthesia network (PRAN) database. Anesth Analg 2015;120(1): 151–6.
[36] McDonnell JG, O'Donnell B, Curley G, et al. The analgesic efficacy of transversus abdominis plane block after abdominal surgery: a prospective randomized controlled trial. Anesth Analg 2007;104(1):193–7.
[37] Fredrickson M, Seal P, Houghton J. Early experience with the transversus abdominis plane block in children. Paediatr Anaesth 2008;18:891–2.
[38] Jagannathan N, Sohn L, Sawardekar A, et al. Unilateral groin surgery in children: will the addition of an ultrasound-guided ilioinguinal nerve block enhance the duration of analgesia of a single-shot caudal block? Paediatr Anaesth 2009;19(1):892–8.
[39] Hannallah RS, Broadman LM, Belman AB, et al. Comparison of caudal and ilioinguinal/iliohypogastric nerve blocks for control of post-orchiopexy pain in pediatric ambulatory surgery. Anesthesiology 1987;66:832–4.

[40] Markham SJ, Tomlinson J, Hain WR. Ilioinguinal nerve block in children. A comparison with caudal block for intra and postoperative analgesia. Anaesthesia 1986;41:1098–103.
[41] Willschke H, Marhofer P, Bösenberg A. Ultrasonography for ilioinguinal/iliohypogastric nerve blocks in children. Br J Anaesth 2005;95(2):226–30.
[42] Ferguson S, Thomas V, Lewis I. The rectus sheath block in paediatric anaesthesia: new indications for an old technique? Paediatr Anaesth 1996;6:463–6.
[43] Willschke H, Bosenberg A, Marhofer P, et al. Ultrasonography-guided rectus sheath block in paediatric anaesthesia: a new approach to an old technique. Br J Anaesth 2006;97: 244–9.
[44] Casati A, Baciarello M, Di Cianni S, et al. Effects of ultrasound guidance on the minimum effective anaesthetic volume required to block the femoral nerve. Br J Anaesth 2007;98: 823–7.
[45] Oberndorfer U, Marhofer P, Bosenberg A, et al. Ultrasonographicguidance for sciatic and femoral nerve blocks in children. Br J Anaesth 2007;98:797–801.
[46] Simion C, Suresh S. Lower extremity peripheral nerve blocks in children. Tech Reg Anesth Pain Manag 2007;11:222–8.
[47] Tsui BC, Ozelsel TJ. Ultrasound-guided anterior sciatic nerve block using a longitudinal approach: "expanding the view". Reg Anesth Pain Med 2008;33:275–6.
[48] Schwemmer U, Markus CK, Greim CA, et al. Sonographic imaging of the sciatic nerve and its division in the popliteal fossa in children. Paediatr Anaesth 2004;14:1005–8.
[49] Tsui B, Suresh S. Ultrasound imaging for regional anesthesia in infants, children, and adolescents: a review of current literature and its application in the practice of extremity and trunk blocks. Anesthesiology 2010;112:473–92.
[50] Shibasaki M, Nakajima Y, Ishii S, et al. Prediction of pediatric endotracheal tube size by ultrasonography. Anesthesiology 2010;113:819–24.
[51] Lakhal K, Delplace X, Cottier JP, et al. The feasibility of ultrasound to assess subglottic diameter. Anesth Analg 2007;104:611–4.
[52] Marciniak B, Fayoux P, Hébrard A, et al. Airway management in children: ultrasonography assessment of tracheal intubation in real time? Anesth Analg 2009;117:461–5.
[53] Dennington D, Vali P, Finer NN, et al. Ultrasound confirmation of endotracheal tube position in neonates. Neonatology 2012;102:185–9.
[54] Stafrace S, Engelhardt T, Teoh WH, et al. Essential ultrasound techniques of the pediatric airway. Paediatr Anaesth 2016;26:122–31.
[55] Sethi A, Nimbalkar A, Patel D, et al. Point of care ultrasonography for position of tip of endotracheal tube in neonates. Indian Pediatr 2014;51:119–21.
[56] Vats A, Worley GA, de Bruyn R, et al. Laryngeal ultrasound to assess vocal fold paralysis in children. J Laryngol Otol 2004;118:429–31.
[57] Fiadjoe JE, Stricker P, Gurnaney H, et al. Ultrasound-guided tracheal intubation: a novel intubation technique. Anesthesiology 2012;117:1389–91.
[58] Kim J, Kim JY, Kim WO, et al. An ultrasound evaluation of laryngeal mask airway position in pediatric patients: an observational study. Anesth Analg 2015;120:427–32.
[59] Wojtczak JA. Submandibular sonography: assessment of hyomental distances and ratio, tongue size, and floor of the mouth musculature using portable sonography. J Ultrasound Med 2012;31:523–8.

Advances in Anesthesia 34 (2016) 85–103

ADVANCES IN ANESTHESIA

Contemporary Perioperative Anesthetic Management of Hepatic Resection

Jonathan A. Wilks, MD, Shannon Hancher-Hodges, MD, Vijaya N.R. Gottumukkala, MD*

Department of Anesthesiology & Perioperative Medicine, The University of Texas MD Anderson Cancer Center, 1400-Unit 409, Holcombe Boulevard, Houston, TX 77030, USA

Keywords

• Liver resection anesthesia • Low CVP anesthesia • Liver ablation anesthesia • Laparoscopic liver surgery • Enhanced recovery

Key points

- Close communication between the surgical and anesthesia teams is a key factor to improve outcomes in liver resections.
- Anesthetic techniques aimed at maintaining low hydrostatic pressures in the inferior vena cava can aid in reducing intraoperative blood loss during parenchymal transection.
- Surgical methods of vascular control to reduce blood loss have hemodynamic consequences that warrant careful preoperative consideration of the anesthesiologist.
- Expanding treatment armamentariums with minimally invasive surgery and ablative therapies have important implications to anesthesia delivery for these new modalities.

INTRODUCTION

Providing anesthesia care for patients undergoing hepatic resection has changed considerably in the past 20 years. Close communication between the surgical and anesthesia teams is a key factor to improve outcomes in these

Disclosure: None of the authors has a relationship with a commercial company that has a direct financial interest in the subject matter or materials discussed in this article or with a company making a competing product.

*Corresponding author. *E-mail address:* vgottumukkala@mdanderson.org

http://dx.doi.org/10.1016/j.aan.2016.07.006

complex procedures. The potential for significant blood loss has always plagued surgeons and anesthesiologists. Surgical and anesthetic techniques have improved significantly the safety profile of hepatic resections. In addition to reviewing these techniques, hepatic anatomy as well as important preoperative considerations are examined. Implications for anesthetic delivery for the expanding treatment armamentarium with laparoscopic techniques and ablative therapies are also discussed.

ANATOMY

To comprehend the extent of hepatic resection, anesthesiologists should have an understanding of the anatomic framework of the liver. The liver can be divided into 8 segments based on the portal supply and hepatic venous drainage; Couinaud's segments retain the name of their initial descriptor in 1954 (Fig. 1) [1,2]. The left, middle, and right hepatic veins serve as 3 vertical divisions; as the portal vein bifurcates into left and right, a horizontal division is created. Couinaud's segments can be understood as they relate to these 3 vertical and 1 horizontal division. Starting from the most superior and left lateral segment II, the segments increase in Roman numeral in a clockwise fashion up to VIII.

The left hepatic vein divides segments II and III from segment IV; segments II and III together are known as the left lateral segment and are divided by the

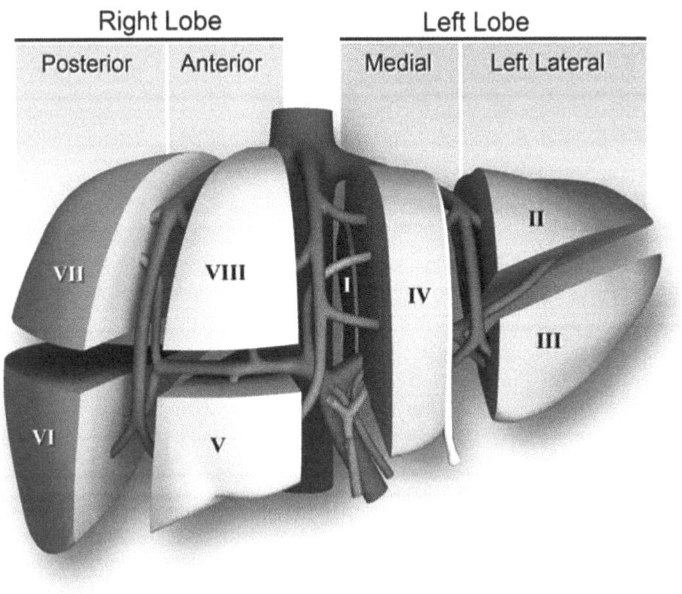

Fig. 1. Segmental liver anatomy. (*From* Sibulesky L. Normal liver anatomy. Clin Liver Dis 2013;2:S1–3.)

portal plane with segmental II superior and III inferior. Segment IV is bounded by the left hepatic vein and middle hepatic vein with divisions above (IVa) and below (IVb) the portal plane. Cantlie's line contains the middle hepatic vein running from the inferior vena cava (IVC) fossa to the gall bladder fossa separating the left and right liver. Lateral (and to the right) to the middle hepatic vein are segments V through VIII. Segments V and VIII are known as the right anterior segment, bounded by the middle and right hepatic veins; the right posterior segment consists of segments VI and VII. Continuing with the clockwise numbering, segments V and VI are inferior to the portal plane, and segments VII and VIII are superior. Each segment has separate portal, biliary, and hepatic arterial branches and drains into the hepatic veins that surround it. Segment I, the caudate lobe, is located posteriorly near the IVC and may receive portal blood from either the left or right portal veins with drainage directly into the IVC via small hepatic veins [3].

The Brisbane 2000 Nomenclature of Hepatic Anatomy and Resections relies on knowledge of Couinaud's segments and has gained tremendous footing in recent years [4]. A left hepatectomy removes segments II, III, and IV; a right hepatectomy removes segments V, VI, VII, and VIII. An extended left hepatectomy adds segments V and VIII to a left hepatectomy, whereas an extended right hepatectomy adds segment IV to a right hepatectomy.

PREOPERATIVE CONSIDERATIONS

In addition to the regular preoperative assessment for any anesthetic (airway, relevant family history for anesthetic complications, and tolerance/complications with previous anesthetics), patients without significant medical comorbidities do not require additional extensive testing, other than blood counts, serum chemistry, and a coagulation profile. Adequate blood product availability will need to be arranged depending on the extent and complex nature of the resection, and preoperative anemia as well as coagulation functions. Additional evaluations are guided by other medical comorbidities, nutritional state, functional status of the patient, and the primary pathology, as well as future remnant of liver.

Cardiovascular

Intraabdominal operations carry an intermediate risk for cardiac adverse events; preoperative cardiac evaluation is guided by a patient's comorbid conditions, risk factors, and functional status [5]. Vascular control mechanisms used in hepatic resections can have profound implications for cardiac patients, necessitating thorough preoperative cardiac assessment of the ability to tolerate the hemodynamic changes with these techniques (Box 1). Patients with limited cardiac reserve may not tolerate pneumoperitoneum of laparoscopic resections with the accompanying marked increase in afterload (wall stress) and decrease in venous return [6].

Portal hypertension associated with advanced liver disease is associated with increased cardiac output with decreased systemic vascular resistance and relative hypovolemia and may be on therapy aimed at reducing symptom burden

Box 1: Techniques used to decrease blood loss

Low central venous pressure anesthesia
Minimizing intravenous fluids (IVF) before hepatic transection
Reverse Trendelenburg positioning
Epidural blockade
Nitroglycerin infusion

Vascular occlusion
Pringle maneuver/portal triad clamping
Anatomic vascular control based on resection
Total hepatic vascular exclusion
Selective hepatic vascular exclusion

Surgical techniques
Cavitron ultrasonic surgical aspirator
Clamp and crush
Surgical staplers
Ultrasonic shears
Sharp Dissection
Two-surgeon technique [102].

(eg, beta-blockers, nitrates, and diuretics for prevention of variceal bleeding and ascites), yet potentially worsen perioperative pathophysiology (further vasodilation and dehydration) [7]. Limited exercise capacity secondary to dyspnea (from ascites, hypoxemia, intrapulmonary shunts, or pulmonary hypertension as opposed to ischemia) may warrant pharmacologic cardiac stress tests [8].

Pulmonary

Pulmonary function tests may guide the anesthesiologist in assessing the reversibility of an obstructive ventilatory defect in symptomatic patients. Decreased room air oxygen saturations may detect patients with hepatopulmonary syndrome: a ventilation/perfusion mismatch owing to increased pulmonary blood flow from capillary dilation with unchanged ventilation and impaired hypoxic pulmonary vasoconstriction [8]. Patients with pulmonary disease are more likely to benefit postoperatively from laparoscopic surgery by avoiding the profound respiratory morbidity associated with open upper abdominal surgery. However, the ventilation changes associated with pneumoperitoneum may present intraoperative challenges in patients with chronic obstructive pulmonary disease. Regional anesthetic techniques (eg, thoracic epidural analgesia or transversus-abdominis-plane blockade) for postoperative pain control in patients with compromised pulmonary function should be considered.

Hepatic

Patients presenting for liver resections may have varying levels of hepatic dysfunction. More important, liver function changes immediately after resection because of decreased liver parenchymal volume as well as postoperative dysfunction of the remnant liver. Anesthetic goals for liver resection should therefore be to avoid exacerbation of preexisting liver dysfunction and to preserve function of the future liver remnant. The sequelae of liver disease can impact every organ system and may have profound implications for anesthetic management, as well as the postoperative course of the patient [9]. Significant effects of portal hypertension include ascites and pleural effusions with impaired respiratory mechanics and aspiration risks, esophageal varices and risk of hemorrhage, and intraabdominal venous collaterals with risk for significant intraoperative blood loss.

Liver anatomy and remnant liver volume are thoroughly evaluated preoperatively by appropriate imaging studies. When needed, preoperative portal vein embolization is performed to increase the size of the remnant liver volume and preserve function [10,11]. Nevertheless, preoperative synthetic liver function is most often surveyed via albumin levels and coagulation studies. Often, determination of resectability may only be obtained intraoperatively. In these cases of possible inoperable anatomy, anesthetic plans should be tailored for potential short operative times.

Patients with hepatocellular carcinoma from underlying chronic hepatitis B infection are more likely to have systemic manifestation of liver dysfunction because of the chronicity of their disease. Metastatic disease may occur in otherwise healthy livers, but underlying parenchymal pathology (eg, steatosis) or neoadjuvant chemotherapy may also adversely impact liver function. Intrahepatic carcinoid tumors may present anesthetic challenges depending on the secretory function of the tumor; octreotide administration may aid in their management [12,13]. Carcinoid crisis may manifest with diarrhea, bronchospasm, dysrhythmias, hypertension, hypotension, and right heart failure.

The presence of cirrhosis is known to increase significantly the postoperative morbidity of abdominal surgery. The Child–Turcotte–Pugh score is 1 way to classify the severity of cirrhosis and is based on serum albumin, bilirubin, prothrombin time, and subjective evaluation of ascites and encephalopathy [14]. The Model for End-stage Liver Disease (MELD) score eliminates ascites and encephalopathy and depends only on bilirubin, creatinine, and international normalized ratio [15]. Not only is MELD used in organ allocation for liver transplantation, several groups have found increased perioperative mortality after hepatic resections for hepatocellular carcinoma in patients with MELD scores of 9 or greater [16,17].

Intrinsic liver disease can result in a bleeding diathesis for several reasons: platelet sequestration and thrombocytopenia from hypersplenism in portal hypertension, coagulopathy from a defect in the synthetic function, and altered activity of the fibrinolytic system. Although lacking validation, thromboelastography may offer guidance in the objective evaluation and management of coagulation abnormalities [9]. Coagulation parameters are not predictive of blood loss or transfusion requirements in hepatic resections [18]. A nomogram created by Sima and colleagues [19] consisting of the number of segments resected, type of lesion, other organ resection, preoperative hemoglobin, and platelets can predict the likelihood of blood transfusion. Evidence from liver transplantation literature argues that correction of abnormal coagulation parameters is unwarranted in patients with severe cirrhosis without obvious symptoms and signs of bleeding [20].

INTRAOPERATIVE MANAGEMENT

Developments in surgical and anesthetic techniques as well as greater appreciation of hepatobiliary surgery as a distinct specialty have likely contributed to overall improvements in perioperative morbidity and mortality. High-volume centers have reported operative mortality of less than 5% [21–25].

Induction of anesthesia is guided by the overall condition of the patient. Rapid sequence induction may be required in patients who have a history of significant ascites or other risk factors for gastric regurgitation. Intravenous access (peripheral or central) sufficient for rapid, large-volume resuscitation is required. In the authors' clinical practice, invasive arterial blood pressure monitoring is used routinely during the procedure. Forced warm-air devices and fluid warmers should be used to guard against hypothermia and its potentiation of a coagulopathy. Benzodiazepines can precipitate hepatic encephalopathy, and the metabolism may be significantly altered, prolonging their effects, questioning the need for routine preoperative anxiolysis with benzodiazepine agents.

General anesthesia is maintained with volatile anesthetics (isoflurane, sevoflurane, desflurane, nitrous oxide), intravenous anesthetics (propofol, dexmedetomidine, ketamine, opiates), or combinations of these. Changes in metabolism in hepatic disease necessitate careful monitoring of the degree of neuromuscular blockade intraoperatively when dosing muscle relaxants. Cisatracurium is often preferred given its predictable Hoffman elimination as well as its lack of significant histamine release. Other short- and intermediate-acting muscle relaxants (atracurium, rocuronium, vecuronium) may also be used safely while bearing in mind their pharmacokinetic and pharmacodynamic profiles [26–29]. Comparing a total intravenous technique (propofol with sufentanil) with a volatile technique (isoflurane with fentanyl) in donor hepatectomy showed no significant advantages of 1 technique over the other [28]. Although no significant clinical difference was found, patients who were administered isoflurane anesthesia had higher postoperative international normalized ratio values and increased liver enzymes compared with patients receiving propofol [30]. A recent randomized trial comparing desflurane with isoflurane in donor hepatectomy revealed higher postoperative international normalized ratio and liver enzymes in patients anesthetized with isoflurane; the clinical significance of this observation in postoperative morbidity was not studied [31]. All volatile anesthetics reduce total hepatic blood flow although the current volatile agents (isoflurane, sevoflurane, desflurane) cause minimal reduction. Less is known about the effects of intravenous anesthetics; however, current evidence suggests minimal effects on hepatic blood flow assuming normal systemic arterial pressure and hemodynamic function [32].

Decreasing blood loss

Liver resections carry an inherent risk of blood loss with surgical dissection of the IVC, portal vein, and hepatic veins and transection of a highly vascularized parenchyma. Furthermore, increased blood loss and perioperative blood transfusions are associated with worse perioperative morbidity and mortality [22,33,34]. As such, significant effort has been focused on reducing intraoperative blood loss.

Roles of both surgeons and anesthesiologists in decreasing blood loss will be discussed (Box 1). Surgeons use various vascular clamps intraoperatively with important anesthetic implications. Similarly, anesthesiologists often use low central venous pressure (CVP) anesthesia until the parenchymal transection is complete.

Pharmacologic interventions aimed at decreasing blood loss (eg, antifibrinolytics) are not frequently studied or used in liver resections; most data are extrapolations from liver transplant literature [35–38]. Similarly, acute normovolemic hemodilution has reduced blood loss and rates of intraoperative transfusions, but current low rates of transfusion question this practice as standard therapy [39–42]. Selective application of acute normovolemic hemodilution may be appropriate in cases expected to lose a large volume of blood.

Low central venous pressure anesthesia

Low CVP anesthesia relies on minimizing hydrostatic pressure in the IVC at the level of the hepatic veins. Blood loss can occur quickly and unexpectedly throughout the operative procedure; surgical dissection of the portal structures, IVC, and hepatic veins represent the earliest opportunity for torrential blood loss. Injury to distended veins, corresponding with increased CVP, can result in profuse bleeding that is difficult to control. A flaccid venous system corresponding with decreased hydrostatic pressure results in a more favorable operative environment for the surgeon.

During parenchymal transection, the surgeon will have temporarily occluded the inflow of blood to the liver (a Pringle maneuver–clamping the portal vein, hepatic artery, and bile duct) while the outflow of blood from the liver (hepatic veins) may not be occluded. Back-bleeding in the parenchyma from the hepatic veins can be not only difficult to control, but can slow transection in the setting of bleeding. Decreased pressure in the IVC at the level of the hepatic veins results in significantly less bleeding during parenchymal transection [39,43–45].

Initial descriptions of this technique come from Memorial Sloan-Kettering Cancer Center and the search for methodologies limiting blood loss [45,46].

Intraoperative CVP as measured in the right atrium would be kept at less than 5 mm Hg until the parenchymal transection was complete; a combination of volatile anesthetic and early intraoperative fluid restriction most commonly accomplished this goal. Intravenous nitroglycerin was used in a minority of cases to reduce CVP. Others report using an epidural blockade with nitroglycerin and dopamine [47]. Johnson and colleagues [43] subsequently reported a strong correlation with increasing retrohepatic IVC pressures and increasing blood loss though suggesting an arbitrary cutoff of less than 6 mm Hg, between 6 and 12 mm Hg, and greater than 13 mm Hg.

Jones and colleagues [44] reported decreased blood loss in patients with parenchymal–transection–CVP of less than 5 cm H_20 (3.7 mm Hg) without description of technique used to obtain this. Others have questioned this arbitrary set point without considering physiologic variability between patients [48]. Indeed, some patients may possess adequate preload with a CVP of 4 mm Hg; more important, all anesthesiologists recognize that this is not the case in all patients.

More recent randomized trials and subsequent metaanalyses have compared low CVP anesthesia by various methods including medications, positional changes, fluid restriction, epidural blockade, and IVC clamping with controls. The conclusions reached in all agree that lower CVP results in decreased blood loss and transfusion requirements; however, no differences between the groups were found in substantive outcomes, that is, morbidity and mortality, with no clear best low CVP technique [39,49–55]. Of significant concern is the possibility of renal injury with a low CVP anesthetic; the largest series (and one of the earliest) does not establish the potential for kidney damage [45]. There remains a lack of evidence demonstrating the safety of 1 technique over another.

Throughout the literature, differences in patient positioning continue to exist. Trendelenburg positioning has been used to decrease the risk of air embolus, improve venous return for renal preservation, and create an ideal situation (as reported by some) for hepatic transection [45,46]. Reverse Trendelenburg positioning has been promoted to decrease CVP and also create an ideal surgical exposure [44,56]. Concern remains for an increased risk for air embolism with reverse Trendelenburg positioning. Air embolism is a known intraoperative complication that can occur not only by opening of a large vein, but also by Venturi effect, with a slightly compressed IVC via small open hepatic veins [44,57]. Moulton and colleagues [58] measured CVP and hepatic venous pressures in 20° head-down, head-up, and supine positions finding no negative intraluminal pressure gradients (a prerequisite for air embolism) with any position suggesting patient positioning does not affect risk of air embolism. Sand and colleagues [56], in a similar experiment, confirmed the findings of Moulton and colleagues that reverse Trendelenburg positioning decreases CVP.

Mirroring our own practice, central venous catheters are not routinely inserted for hepatic resections [8,59,60]. Because CVP monitoring has drastically decreased in our institution, creating an environment (low hydrostatic IVC pressures) that minimizes hepatic venous bleeding relies on a volume-sparing anesthetic (preoperatively until transection is complete), reverse Trendelenburg positioning, and continued trust and communication between surgical and anesthesia teams.

Surgical techniques

J.H. Pringle [61] was the first to describe methods to decrease hemorrhage from the liver by occluding the vascular inflow. Portal triad clamping, also known as hepatic pedicle clamping and the Pringle maneuver, remains widely used in liver resections. Surgeons now have multiple different methods of vascular control in their armamentarium to assist in reducing blood loss during liver resections, each with different anesthetic implications.

The Pringle maneuver results in characteristic hemodynamic changes: increased blood pressure and systemic vascular resistance with decreased cardiac output (Table 1) [62]. These hemodynamic alterations are expected to return to normal shortly after releasing the occlusion. A prospective randomized trial revealed that, although continuous portal triad clamping allows for decreased blood loss, intermittent portal triad clamping results in less hepatic injury as measured by postoperative laboratory values and fewer cases of postoperative liver failure [63].

Vascular control may also be obtained at more selective levels as indicated for the intended resection. Hilar dissection is required to delineate the appropriate hepatic arterial and portal venous branches; this is a more complicated pretransection technique. Advantages include significantly fewer hemodynamic changes, ischemic demarcation for transection limits, and preservation of remnant parenchyma with no exposure to ischemia during transection [53,64–66].

Total hepatic vascular exclusion involves occluding the infrahepatic IVC, suprahepatic IVC, and portal triad. This technique is often reserved for tumors close to the IVC or hepatic veins. Anesthetic management of total hepatic vascular exclusion is vastly different from any other liver resection. Volume preloading when appropriate (maintaining euvolemia) is required before the caval clamping to prevent a sudden decrease in cardiac output; heart rate and systemic vascular resistance will increase substantially. A test clamping period should be attempted before transection to determine physiologic tolerance.

Table 1
Characteristic hemodynamic changes with techniques used to decrease blood loss

	Mean arterial pressure	Heart rate	Cardiac output	Systemic vascular resistance	Central venous pressure
Trendelenburg	↑	↓	↑	↑/↓	↑
Reverse Trendelenburg	↓	↑	↓	↑/↓	↓
Pringle	↑	↑	↓	↑	↓
Total vascular occlusion	↓	↑	↓	↑	↓

Control of the hepatic outflow via the hepatic veins at the suprahepatic IVC provides another mechanism to prevent back-bleeding during transection; occlusion of the hepatic veins (all or selective) has been described in conjunction with the Pringle maneuver as well as selective inflow occlusion [64,65,67–70]. Selective hepatic vascular exclusion (portal triad and hepatic vein isolation) allows isolation from all inflow and nearly all outflow with preservation of caval flow avoiding the hemodynamic consequences of total hepatic vascular exclusion [69]. Selective hepatic vascular exclusion may also be used when the CVP is thought to be too high despite efforts to lower it [71].

Several metaanalyses have attempted to determine superiority among the different surgical techniques used during hepatic resections to decrease blood loss. Richardson and colleagues [72] found no difference between portal triad clamping and other forms of vascular control. A recent network metaanalysis concluded that continuous vascular occlusion results in decreased blood loss and transfusion requirements; given the small number of studies included, no conclusion regarding which method of vascular occlusion was best could be made [73]. Simillis and colleagues [73] also searched for superiority of the surgical methods of transection (eg, clamp-crush, Cavitron ultrasonic surgical aspirator, sharp dissection, ultrasonic shears, etc) and found none.

LAPAROSCOPIC LIVER RESECTION

Recent advances in surgical techniques and medical technology combined with a focus on patient-centered outcomes have led to greater adoption of minimally invasive techniques across the surgical practice. Minilaparotomy, laparoscopy, and robotic-assisted surgery are increasingly being adopted in liver surgery. Robotic-assisted surgery has been gaining some popularity because it overcomes some of the limitations of laparoscopic surgery, such as loss of 3-dimensional vision, reduced surgeon hand–eye coordination, and instrument articulation. However, lack of haptic feedback, difficulties encountered in robot docking, cost issues, and the need for an additional experienced surgeon for emergency conversion remain limitations for widespread adoption. In addition to the specific perioperative considerations for open liver surgery, critical issues for the anesthesiologist during laparoscopic and robotic procedures include factors related to the physiologic consequences of pneumoperitoneum, patient positioning, restricted vascular access to the patient in an emergency, and venous gas embolism. A general trend toward shorter duration of hospital stays has been noted, but institutional and geographic differences make large-scale analyses difficult [74].

The different techniques of laparoscopic liver resections vary in the size of the incision used to assist with surgery [75]. Pure laparoscopic resection only requires a Pfannenstiel incision to remove the specimen in addition to the port sites. Hand-assisted laparoscopy uses a small incision for a hand gel-port and eventual specimen removal. Laparoscopic-assisted hepatectomy involves a minilaparotomy for parenchymal transection after laparoscopic dissection.

Pneumoperitoneum has significant ventilatory effects: increasing peak inspiratory pressures by 35%, decreasing pulmonary compliance by as much as 27%, decreased functional residual capacity, and decreased lung volumes over time favoring atelectasis [76]. Intraperitoneal insufflation results in predictable hemodynamic changes of increased mean arterial pressure and systemic vascular resistance without significant changes in heart rate [77]. Increased CVP values reported with pneumoperitoneum do not necessarily indicate increased central blood volume. An increased intrathoracic–intraabdominal IVC gradient with insufflation results in a brief increase followed by a decrease in cardiac filling, suggesting increased CVP values come from transmitted intrathoracic pressures [77–80]. Reverse Trendelenburg positioning is common for laparoscopic hepatic resections [66]. A further reduction in preload can be expected upon changing to a reverse Trendelenburg position [77]. Other positions used in laparoscopic liver resections include decubitus and the French position, with the surgeon standing between legs in stirrups for improved ergonomics with occasional thoracoscopic exposure for posterior–superior lesions. Arms are frequently tucked, emphasizing the importance of obtaining adequate vascular access and monitoring before positioning.

Although heart rate does not predictably change during pneumoperitoneum, occasional vagal responses with insufflation can result in hemodynamically significant bradycardia requiring treatment. Absorbed carbon dioxide resulting in hypercarbia can cause sympathetic nervous system activation with increased heart rate, blood pressure, and myocardial contractility [81,82].

The changes in blood pressure and systemic vascular resistance that occur with pneumoperitoneum mirror those with hepatic pedicle clamping, raising concern about potential additive effects. Comparing hemodynamic variables related to hepatic pedicle clamping in laparoscopic resections with that in open resections revealed similar patterns and no differences between groups [83]. The hemodynamic changes associated with hepatic pedicle clamping in both open and laparoscopic resections are well-tolerated [83–85]. Also of concern is the potential for air embolism with pneumoperitoneum; Farges and colleagues [85] found no increased risk of air embolism during laparoscopic resections compared with open procedures.

Standard preoperative fasting requirements before elective surgery may create fluid deficits in patients at the time of induction of anesthesia, and continued volume sparing remains important in minimizing blood loss during the parenchymal transection by minimizing hydrostatic IVC pressures to reduce hepatic venous bleeding. The additive effects of intravenous fluid restriction before parenchymal transection, reverse Trendelenburg positioning, and pneumoperitoneum during laparoscopic liver resection decrease venous return significantly, which needs to be anticipated (Table 2). Young and otherwise healthy patients may be able to tolerate this hypovolemic state without significant intervention; however, most patients will require goal-directed or intervention-assessed volume administration during the preresection period to sustain perfusion pressure [45].

Table 2
Preload changes in laparoscopic liver resections

Intervention	Effect on cardiac preload
Minimizing IVF until transection complete	Decrease
Reverse Trendelenburg positioning	Decrease
Pneumoperitoneum	Decrease

ABLATIVE THERAPIES

Not all patients with liver lesions are candidates for hepatic resection; significant tumor burden, anatomic considerations, or preoperative liver function may preclude attempts at resection. Liver tumor ablation involves the direct application of energy or chemicals to illicit cell death of the hepatic lesion while minimizing injury to normal surrounding parenchyma. Ablations are performed commonly for patients with hepatocellular carcinoma and metastases from colorectal cancer. Chemical methods include direct ethanol injection and transarterial chemoembolization. Energy-based therapies can be classified as thermal (hot or cold) or nonthermal (Table 3).

Radiofrequency ablation is perhaps the most well-studied technique; energy is applied via electrodes in the 375 to 500 KHz range [86]. Radiofrequency ablation is suited best for tumors smaller than 3 cm and those that are not close to vasculature if larger than 3 mm; tissue heating causes denatured proteins resulting in cell death [87]. Heat applied near vasculature (a continuous flow of normothermic blood) dissipates in this perivascular space; this heat sink effect is responsible for incomplete ablation of perivascular tumors [88].

Microwave ablation applies energy in the 915 MHz to 2.45 GHz range to generate high temperatures over a short time. Microwave ablation overcomes some of the shortcomings of radiofrequency ablation in its ability to treat tumors larger than 3 cm with less of a concern over the heat sink effect [86,89].

Cryoablation involves the application of cold freezing temperatures or freeze–thaw cycles to disrupt cell membranes resulting in cell death. Advantages include the ability to follow the ice ball formation with imaging and decreased pain. Cryoshock (an inflammatory response) occurring after the

Table 3
Ablation therapies

Technique	Energy	Advantages	Disadvantages
Radiofrequency ablation	Thermal (heat)	Lesions <3 cm	Heat sink effect
Microwave ablation	Thermal (heat)	Lesions >3 cm Less heat sink	Difficult to control rapid heating zone
Cryoablation	Thermal (cold)	Follow ice-ball formation	Lack of cautery effects
Irreversible electroporation	Nonthermal (electric)	Preserves normal structural environment	Potential cardiac dysrhythmias General anesthesia

procedure is a potential disadvantage, as well as the lack of hemostatic effects present in high-energy therapies [86].

Delivering anesthesia for liver ablation therapies can range from local anesthetics and light sedation to general anesthesia depending on the method of application, provider experience, and patient selection. Probes may be inserted percutaneously or directly into liver parenchyma with an open incision and ultrasound guidance. Heat therapies are often associated with discomfort, which may necessitate a deeper anesthetic.

Irreversible electroporation

Irreversible electroporation (IRE) is a relatively new ablative therapy that carries very specific anesthetic considerations deserving special attention (Table 4). Multiple high-voltage electrical pulses applied within a lesion disrupt cellular membranes irreversibly (with sufficient voltage) with subsequent apoptosis [87,90]. A significant advantage of IRE is the ability to apply energy to a lesion without causing damage to the surrounding structural environment rich in extracellular collagen (ie, vasculature, bile ducts, and gallbladder) and without the concern for a heat sink effect [91,92].

Pulsatile delivery of high-voltage electrical energy has the potential to cause significant harm to patients. In the percutaneous delivery of IRE, the electrodes are inserted through the abdominal wall musculature; activation of the electrodes would result in significant muscle contraction without the use of muscle relaxants. For this reason, IRE cases are performed under general anesthesia with complete muscle relaxation [92].

Transmitted electrical energy to the heart has the potential to cause dysrhythmias. In one of the initial descriptions of anesthetic delivery for IRE, 25% of patients (7 of 28) developed brief episodes of ventricular tachycardia that were temporally related to treatment pulses [93]. Although Ball and colleagues [93] were unable to determine safe distances for cardiac transmission (ie, dysrhythmias occurred in patients undergoing IRE for lesions in the lungs, liver, and kidney), they commented that the most significant dysrhythmia occurred while treating a hepatic lesion abutting the diaphragm and close to the inferior border of the heart. The use of devices that synchronize electrical pulses during the absolute refractory period of the heart reduces the likelihood that pulses will generate a ventricular action potential, but dysrhythmias continue to be reported [92,94].

Table 4
Anesthetic requirements for irreversible electroporation

General anesthesia	Required with the use of neuromuscular relaxation
Complete neuromuscular relaxation	Avoids significant muscle contractions during procedure
Cardiac synchronization of electrical pulses	Reduces likelihood of cardiac conduction and potential for severe dysrhythmias

Another theoretic risk of pulsed electrical energy is induction of epileptic activity in patients with decreased thresholds. Cardiac synchronization (ie, pulses set at rates lower than the frequencies associated with seizure induction) is thought to reduce this risk, and Nielsen and colleagues [92] were not able to demonstrate cerebral activity during electrical pulses during IRE.

ENHANCED RECOVERY

Enhanced recovery protocols have been used recently in both laparoscopic and open liver resections [95–100]. These protocols are evidence-based perioperative clinical pathways developed to accelerate functional recovery of patients undergoing operations. The goal is to reduce the incidence of postoperative symptoms and complications (through the use of multimodal opioid-sparing pain management strategies), accelerate functional recovery, increase patient satisfaction and safety after discharge with no increase in readmission rates or postdischarge complications, and reduce the duration of hospital stay. Components of enhanced recovery span multiple disciplines and include patient education and engagement, opiate-sparing anesthesia and analgesia, avoidance of hypervolemia, avoidance of bowel and bladder tubes, early ambulation, diet advancement, and early ambulation [101]. Multimodal regimens currently include celecoxib, acetaminophen, and gabapentinoids, as well as local anesthetic blockade in wound infiltration, field blocks, or thoracic epidural catheters.

Multiple centers have now published their experience demonstrating safety with implementation of enhanced recovery protocols and improvement in durations of stay for both open and laparoscopic liver resections [95–97,100,101]. Furthermore, our institution has demonstrated an acceleration in the time between surgery and subsequent adjuvant therapy, that is, return to intended oncologic therapy [101].

Enhanced surveillance, advancements in radiographic imaging, incorporating neoadjuvant therapy in treatment care strategies, and improvements in surgical and perioperative care have resulted in improvements in survival after hepatic resection for metastatic colorectal cancers in high volume centers. However, perioperative care among centers that perform liver resections still varies substantially. A better understanding of the perioperative considerations of liver surgery by the anesthesiology community, and effective intraoperative communication between the surgical and anesthesiology teams will enhance surgical and perioperative outcomes. Developing multidisciplinary patient-centered perioperative care pathways to minimize symptom burden, enhance functional recovery, rapid rescue from postoperative complications, and efforts to improve return to intended oncologic therapy rates have the potential to improve oncological outcomes.

References

[1] Couinaud C. Liver lobes and segments: notes on the anatomical architecture and surgery of the liver. Presse Med 1954;62(33):709–12 [in French].
[2] Sibulesky L. Normal liver anatomy. Clin Liver Dis 2013;2:S1–3.

[3] Abdalla EK, Vauthey JN, Couinaud C. The caudate lobe of the liver: implications of embryology and anatomy for surgery. Surg Oncol Clin N Am 2002;11(4):835–48.

[4] Strasberg SM, Phillips C. Use and dissemination of the Brisbane 2000 nomenclature of liver anatomy and resections. Ann Surg 2013;257(3):377–82.

[5] American College of Cardiology/American Heart Association Task Force on Practice Guidelines (Writing Committee to Revise the 2002 Guidelines on Perioperative Cardiovascular Evaluation for Noncardiac Surgery), American Society of Echocardiography, American Society of Nuclear Cardiology, et al. ACC/AHA 2007 guidelines on perioperative cardiovascular evaluation and care for noncardiac surgery: executive summary: a report of the American College of Cardiology/American Heart Association Task Force on Practice Guidelines (Writing Committee to Revise the 2002 Guidelines on Perioperative Cardiovascular Evaluation for Noncardiac Surgery). Anesth Analg 2008;106(3):685–712.

[6] Sharma KC, Kabinoff G, Ducheine Y, et al. Laparoscopic surgery and its potential for medical complications. Heart Lung 1997;26(1):52–64 [quiz: 65–7].

[7] Vaughan RB, Chin-Dusting JP. Current pharmacotherapy in the management of cirrhosis: focus on the hyperdynamic circulation. Expert Opin Pharmacother 2003;4(5):625–37.

[8] Redai I, Emond J, Brentjens T. Anesthetic considerations during liver surgery. Surg Clin North Am 2004;84(2):401–11.

[9] Kiamanesh D, Rumley J, Moitra VK. Monitoring and managing hepatic disease in anaesthesia. Br J Anaesth 2013;111(Suppl 1):i50–61.

[10] Abdalla EK, Barnett CC, Doherty D, et al. Extended hepatectomy in patients with hepatobiliary malignancies with and without preoperative portal vein embolization. Arch Surg 2002;137(6):675–80 [discussion: 680–1].

[11] Kishi Y, Abdalla EK, Chun YS, et al. Three hundred and one consecutive extended right hepatectomies: evaluation of outcome based on systematic liver volumetry. Ann Surg 2009;250(4):540–8.

[12] Kinney MA, Warner ME, Nagorney DM, et al. Perianaesthetic risks and outcomes of abdominal surgery for metastatic carcinoid tumours. Br J Anaesth 2001;87(3):447–52.

[13] Massimino K, Harrskog O, Pommier S, et al. Octreotide LAR and bolus octreotide are insufficient for preventing intraoperative complications in carcinoid patients. J Surg Oncol 2013;107(8):842–6.

[14] Pugh RN, Murray-Lyon IM, Dawson JL, et al. Transection of the oesophagus for bleeding oesophageal varices. Br J Surg 1973;60(8):646–9.

[15] Malinchoc M, Kamath PS, Gordon FD, et al. A model to predict poor survival in patients undergoing transjugular intrahepatic portosystemic shunts. Hepatology 2000;31(4):864–71.

[16] Cucchetti A, Ercolani G, Vivarelli M, et al. Impact of Model for End-stage Liver Disease (MELD) score on prognosis after hepatectomy for hepatocellular carcinoma on cirrhosis. Liver Transpl 2006;12(6):966–71.

[17] Teh SH, Christein J, Donohue J, et al. Hepatic resection of hepatocellular carcinoma in patients with cirrhosis: Model of End-Stage Liver Disease (MELD) score predicts perioperative mortality. J Gastrointest Surg 2005;9(9):1207–15 [discussion: 1215].

[18] McNally SJ, Revie EJ, Massie LJ, et al. Factors in perioperative care that determine blood loss in liver surgery. HPB (Oxford) 2012;14(4):236–41.

[19] Sima CS, Jarnagin WR, Fong Y, et al. Predicting the risk of perioperative transfusion for patients undergoing elective hepatectomy. Ann Surg 2009;250(6):914–21.

[20] Massicotte L, Beaulieu D, Thibeault L, et al. Coagulation defects do not predict blood product requirements during liver transplantation. Transplantation 2008;85(7):956–62.

[21] Belghiti J, Hiramatsu K, Benoist S, et al. Seven hundred forty-seven hepatectomies in the 1990s: an update to evaluate the actual risk of liver resection. J Am Coll Surg 2000;191(1):38–46.

[22] Jarnagin WR, Gonen M, Fong Y, et al. Improvement in perioperative outcome after hepatic resection: analysis of 1,803 consecutive cases over the past decade. Ann Surg 2002;236(4):397–406 [discussion: 406–7].
[23] Tsao JI, Loftus JP, Nagorney DM, et al. Trends in morbidity and mortality of hepatic resection for malignancy. A matched comparative analysis. Ann Surg 1994;220(2):199–205.
[24] Fong Y, Fortner J, Sun RL, et al. Clinical score for predicting recurrence after hepatic resection for metastatic colorectal cancer: analysis of 1001 consecutive cases. Ann Surg 1999;230(3):309–18 [discussion: 318–21].
[25] Mullen JT, Ribero D, Reddy SK, et al. Hepatic insufficiency and mortality in 1,059 noncirrhotic patients undergoing major hepatectomy. J Am Coll Surg 2007;204(5):854–62 [discussion: 862–4].
[26] Martucci G, Burgio G, Spada M, et al. Anesthetic management of totally robotic right lobe living-donor hepatectomy: new tools ask for perioperative care. Eur Rev Med Pharmacol Sci 2013;17(14):1974–7.
[27] Niemann CU, Feiner J, Behrends M, et al. Central venous pressure monitoring during living right donor hepatectomy. Liver Transpl 2007;13(2):266–71.
[28] Rabie M, Negmi H, Hammad Y, et al. Living donor hepatectomy (LDH)–comparative study between two different anesthetic techniques. Middle East J Anesthesiol 2006;18(4):743–56.
[29] Siniscalchi A, Begliomini B, Matteo G, et al. Intraoperative effects of combined versus general anesthesia during major liver surgery. Minerva Anestesiol 2003;69(12):885–95.
[30] Ozgul U, Ucar M, Erdogan MA, et al. Effects of isoflurane and propofol on hepatic and renal functions and coagulation profile after right hepatectomy in living donors. Transplant Proc 2013;45(3):966–70.
[31] Toprak HI, Sahin T, Aslan S, et al. Effects of desflurane and isoflurane on hepatic and renal functions and coagulation profile during donor hepatectomy. Transplant Proc 2012;44(6):1635–9.
[32] Rothenberg DM, O'Connor CJ, Tuman KJ. Anesthesia and the hepatobiliary system. In: Miller RD, editor. Miller's anesthesia. 7th edition. Philadelphia: Churchill Livingstone/Elsevier; 2010. p. 2135–54.
[33] Jamieson GG, Corbel L, Campion JP, et al. Major liver resection without a blood transfusion: is it a realistic objective? Surgery 1992;112(1):32–6.
[34] Nagorney DM, van Heerden JA, Ilstrup DM, et al. Primary hepatic malignancy: surgical management and determinants of survival. Surgery 1989;106(4):740–8 [discussion: 748–9].
[35] Alkozai EM, Lisman T, Porte RJ. Bleeding in liver surgery: prevention and treatment. Clin Liver Dis 2009;13(1):145–54.
[36] Gurusamy KS, Li J, Sharma D, et al. Pharmacological interventions to decrease blood loss and blood transfusion requirements for liver resection. Cochrane Database Syst Rev 2009;(4):CD008085.
[37] Lentschener C, Benhamou D, Mercier FJ, et al. Aprotinin reduces blood loss in patients undergoing elective liver resection. Anesth Analg 1997;84(4):875–81.
[38] Wu CC, Ho WM, Cheng SB, et al. Perioperative parenteral tranexamic acid in liver tumor resection: a prospective randomized trial toward a "blood transfusion"-free hepatectomy. Ann Surg 2006;243(2):173–80.
[39] Gurusamy KS, Li J, Vaughan J, et al. Cardiopulmonary interventions to decrease blood loss and blood transfusion requirements for liver resection. Cochrane Database Syst Rev 2012;(5):CD007338.
[40] Jarnagin WR, Gonen M, Maithel SK, et al. A prospective randomized trial of acute normovolemic hemodilution compared to standard intraoperative management in patients undergoing major hepatic resection. Ann Surg 2008;248(3):360–9.
[41] Maithel SK, Jarnagin WR. Adjuncts to liver surgery: is acute normovolemic hemodilution useful for major hepatic resections? Adv Surg 2009;43:259–68.

[42] Matot I, Scheinin O, Jurim O, et al. Effectiveness of acute normovolemic hemodilution to minimize allogeneic blood transfusion in major liver resections. Anesthesiology 2002;97(4):794–800.
[43] Johnson M, Mannar R, Wu AV. Correlation between blood loss and inferior vena caval pressure during liver resection. Br J Surg 1998;85(2):188–90.
[44] Jones RM, Moulton CE, Hardy KJ. Central venous pressure and its effect on blood loss during liver resection. Br J Surg 1998;85(8):1058–60.
[45] Melendez JA, Arslan V, Fischer ME, et al. Perioperative outcomes of major hepatic resections under low central venous pressure anesthesia: blood loss, blood transfusion, and the risk of postoperative renal dysfunction. J Am Coll Surg 1998;187(6):620–5.
[46] Cunningham JD, Fong Y, Shriver C, et al. One hundred consecutive hepatic resections. Blood loss, transfusion, and operative technique. Arch Surg 1994;129(10):1050–6.
[47] Rees M, Plant G, Wells J, et al. One hundred and fifty hepatic resections: evolution of technique towards bloodless surgery. Br J Surg 1996;83(11):1526–9.
[48] Bhattacharya S, Jackson DJ, Beard CI, et al. Central venous pressure and its effects on blood loss during liver resection. Br J Surg 1999;86(2):282–3.
[49] Hughes MJ, Ventham NT, Harrison EM, et al. Central venous pressure and liver resection: a systematic review and meta-analysis. HPB (Oxford) 2015;17(10):863–71.
[50] Li Z, Sun YM, Wu FX, et al. Controlled low central venous pressure reduces blood loss and transfusion requirements in hepatectomy. World J Gastroenterol 2014;20(1):303–9.
[51] Wang WD, Liang LJ, Huang XQ, et al. Low central venous pressure reduces blood loss in hepatectomy. World J Gastroenterol 2006;12(6):935–9.
[52] Kato M, Kubota K, Kita J, et al. Effect of infra-hepatic inferior vena cava clamping on bleeding during hepatic dissection: a prospective, randomized, controlled study. World J Gastroenterol 2008;32(6):1082–7.
[53] Figueras J, Llado L, Ruiz D, et al. Complete versus selective portal triad clamping for minor liver resections: a prospective randomized trial. Ann Surg 2005;241(4):582–90.
[54] Rahbari NN, Koch M, Zimmermann JB, et al. Infrahepatic inferior vena cava clamping for reduction of central venous pressure and blood loss during hepatic resection: a randomized controlled trial. Ann Surg 2011;253(6):1102–10.
[55] Zhu P, Lau WY, Chen YF, et al. Randomized clinical trial comparing infrahepatic inferior vena cava clamping with low central venous pressure in complex liver resections involving the Pringle manoeuvre. Br J Surg 2012;99(6):781–8.
[56] Sand L, Rizell M, Houltz E, et al. Effect of patient position and PEEP on hepatic, portal and central venous pressures during liver resection. Acta Anaesthesiol Scand 2011;55(9):1106–12.
[57] Hatano Y, Murakawa M, Segawa H, et al. Venous air embolism during hepatic resection. Anesthesiology 1990;73(6):1282–5.
[58] Moulton CA, Chui AK, Mann D, et al. Does patient position during liver surgery influence the risk of venous air embolism? Am J Surg 2001;181(4):366–7.
[59] Franco D. Liver surgery has become simpler. Eur J Anaesthesiol 2002;19(11):777–9.
[60] Lentschener C, Ozier Y. Anaesthesia for elective liver resection: some points should be revisited. Eur J Anaesthesiol 2002;19(11):780–8.
[61] Pringle JH. V. Notes on the arrest of hepatic hemorrhage due to trauma. Ann Surg 1908;48(4):541–9.
[62] Delva E, Camus Y, Paugam C, et al. Hemodynamic effects of portal triad clamping in humans. Anesth Analg 1987;66(9):864–8.
[63] Belghiti J, Noun R, Malafosse R, et al. Continuous versus intermittent portal triad clamping for liver resection: a controlled study. Ann Surg 1999;229(3):369–75.
[64] Abdalla EK, Noun R, Belghiti J. Hepatic vascular occlusion: which technique? Surg Clin North Am 2004;84(2):563–85.

[65] Moug SJ, Smith D, Leen E, et al. Selective continuous vascular occlusion and perioperative fluid restriction in partial hepatectomy. Outcomes in 101 consecutive patients. Eur J Surg Oncol 2007;33(8):1036–41.
[66] Yan CY, Cai XJ, Wang YF. Effect of selective inflow occlusion on hemodynamic conditions during laparoscopic left hemihepatectomy effect of selective inflow occlusion on hemodynamic conditions during laparoscopic left hemihepatectomy. Hepatogastroenterology 2012;59(114):501–4.
[67] Smyrniotis VE, Kostopanagiotou GG, Contis JC, et al. Selective hepatic vascular exclusion versus Pringle maneuver in major liver resections: prospective study. World J Surg 2003;27(7):765–9.
[68] Zhou W, Li A, Pan Z, et al. Selective hepatic vascular exclusion and Pringle maneuver: a comparative study in liver resection. Eur J Surg Oncol 2008;34(1):49–54.
[69] Cherqui D, Malassagne B, Colau PI, et al. Hepatic vascular exclusion with preservation of the caval flow for liver resections. Ann Surg 1999;230(1):24–30.
[70] Chouillard EK, Gumbs AA, Cherqui D. Vascular clamping in liver surgery: physiology, indications and techniques. Ann Surg Innov Res 2010;4:2.
[71] Tympa A, Theodoraki K, Tsaroucha A, et al. Anesthetic considerations in hepatectomies under hepatic vascular control. HPB Surg 2012;2012:720754.
[72] Richardson AJ, Laurence JM, Lam VW. Portal triad clamping versus other methods of vascular control in liver resection: a systematic review and meta-analysis. HPB (Oxford) 2012;14(6):355–64.
[73] Simillis C, Li T, Vaughan J, et al. A Cochrane systematic review and network meta-analysis comparing treatment strategies aiming to decrease blood loss during liver resection. Int J Surg 2015;23(Pt A):128–36.
[74] Reddy SK, Tsung A, Geller DA. Laparoscopic liver resection. World J Surg 2011;35(7):1478–86.
[75] Lin NC, Nitta H, Wakabayashi G. Laparoscopic major hepatectomy: a systematic literature review and comparison of 3 techniques. Ann Surg 2013;257(2):205–13.
[76] Valenza F, Chevallard G, Fossali T, et al. Management of mechanical ventilation during laparoscopic surgery. Best Pract Res Clin Anaesthesiol 2010;24(2):227–41.
[77] Joris JL, Noirot DP, Legrand MJ, et al. Hemodynamic changes during laparoscopic cholecystectomy. Anesth Analg 1993;76(5):1067–71.
[78] Giebler RM, Behrends M, Steffens T, et al. Intraperitoneal and retroperitoneal carbon dioxide insufflation evoke different effects on caval vein pressure gradients in humans: evidence for the starling resistor concept of abdominal venous return. Anesthesiology 2000;92(6):1568–80.
[79] Hein HA, Joshi GP, Ramsay MA, et al. Hemodynamic changes during laparoscopic cholecystectomy in patients with severe cardiac disease. J Clin Anesth 1997;9(4):261–5.
[80] O'Malley C, Cunningham AJ. Physiologic changes during laparoscopy. Anesthesiol Clin North America 2001;19(1):1–19.
[81] Gerges FJ, Kanazi GE, Jabbour-Khoury SI. Anesthesia for laparoscopy: a review. J Clin Anesth 2006;18(1):67–78.
[82] Nguyen NT, Wolfe BM. The physiologic effects of pneumoperitoneum in the morbidly obese. Ann Surg 2005;241(2):219–26.
[83] Decailliot F, Cherqui D, Leroux B, et al. Effects of portal triad clamping on haemodynamic conditions during laparoscopic liver resection. Br J Anaesth 2001;87(3):493–6.
[84] Decailliot F, Streich B, Heurtematte Y, et al. Hemodynamic effects of portal triad clamping with and without pneumoperitoneum: an echocardiographic study. Anesth Analg 2005;100(3):617–22.
[85] Farges O, Jagot P, Kirstetter P, et al. Prospective assessment of the safety and benefit of laparoscopic liver resections. J Hepatobiliary Pancreat Surg 2002;9(2):242–8.

[86] Lencioni R, de Baere T, Martin RC, et al. Image-guided ablation of malignant liver tumors: recommendations for clinical validation of novel thermal and non-thermal technologies - a western perspective. Liver Cancer 2015;4(4):208–14.
[87] Narayanan G, Froud T, Suthar R, et al. Irreversible electroporation of hepatic malignancy. Semin Intervent Radiol 2013;30(1):67–73.
[88] Narayanan G. Irreversible electroporation for treatment of liver cancer. Gastroenterol Hepatol (N Y) 2011;7(5):313–6.
[89] Lubner MG, Brace CL, Ziemlewicz TJ, et al. Microwave ablation of hepatic malignancy. Semin Intervent Radiol 2013;30(1):56–66.
[90] Scheffer HJ, Nielsen K, de Jong MC, et al. Irreversible electroporation for nonthermal tumor ablation in the clinical setting: a systematic review of safety and efficacy. J Vasc Interv Radiol 2014;25(7):997–1011 [quiz: 1011].
[91] Hosein PJ, Echenique A, Loaiza-Bonilla A, et al. Percutaneous irreversible electroporation for the treatment of colorectal cancer liver metastases with a proposal for a new response evaluation system. J Vasc Interv Radiol 2014;25(8):1233–9.e2.
[92] Nielsen K, Scheffer HJ, Vieveen JM, et al. Anaesthetic management during open and percutaneous irreversible electroporation. Br J Anaesth 2014;113(6):985–92.
[93] Ball C, Thomson KR, Kavnoudias H. Irreversible electroporation: a new challenge in "out of operating theater" anesthesia. Anesth Analg 2010;110(5):1305–9.
[94] Deodhar A, Dickfeld T, Single GW, et al. Irreversible electroporation near the heart: ventricular arrhythmias can be prevented with ECG synchronization. AJR Am J Roentgenol 2011;196(3):W330–5.
[95] Schultz NA, Larsen PN, Klarskov B, et al. Evaluation of a fast-track programme for patients undergoing liver resection. Br J Surg 2013;100(1):138–43.
[96] Stoot JH, van Dam RM, Busch OR, et al. The effect of a multimodal fast-track programme on outcomes in laparoscopic liver surgery: a multicentre pilot study. HPB (Oxford) 2009;11(2):140–4.
[97] He F, Lin X, Xie F, et al. The effect of enhanced recovery program for patients undergoing partial laparoscopic hepatectomy of liver cancer. Clin Transl Oncol 2015;17(9): 694–701.
[98] Hughes MJ, McNally S, Wigmore SJ. Enhanced recovery following liver surgery: a systematic review and meta-analysis. HPB (Oxford) 2014;16(8):699–706.
[99] Jones C, Kelliher L, Dickinson M, et al. Randomized clinical trial on enhanced recovery versus standard care following open liver resection. Br J Surg 2013;100(8):1015–24.
[100] Savikko J, Ilmakunnas M, Makisalo H, et al. Enhanced recovery protocol after liver resection. Br J Surg 2015;102(12):1526–32.
[101] Day RW, Cleeland CS, Wang XS, et al. Patient-reported outcomes accurately measure the value of an enhanced recovery program in liver surgery. J Am Coll Surg 2015;221(6): 1023–30.e1-2.
[102] Day RW, Brudvik KW, Vauthey JN, et al. Advances in hepatectomy technique: toward zero transfusions in the modern era of liver surgery. Surgery 2016;159(3):793–801.

Advances in Anesthesia 34 (2016) 105–115

ADVANCES IN ANESTHESIA

Role of Regional Anesthesia and Analgesia on Perioperative Outcomes in Patients with Hip Fracture

Bridget Perrin Pulos, MD, Jiabin Liu, MD, PhD,
Mark D. Neuman, MD, MS, Nabil M. Elkassabany, MD, MSCE*

Department of Anesthesiology and Critical Care, Perelman School of Medicine, University of Pennsylvania, Philadelphia, PA, USA

Keywords

• Hip fracture • Orthopedic trauma • Geriatric fractures • Anesthesia
• Postoperative • Pain management • Patients' outcomes

Key points

- Perioperative management of patients with hip fracture may impact patients' outcomes. Whether neuraxial anesthesia improves patient outcomes is still debated.
- This manuscript summarizes evidence supporting or refuting any advantage for regional anesthesia, specifically reviewing evidence for the effect of regional anesthesia on mortality, complications, and health care cost.
- Peripheral nerve blocks are becoming more popular option to integrate into the pain management protocol in this patient population.
- Peripheral nerve blocks may offer some advantage in terms of using less opioids and potentially less side effects.
- The current article reviews the different techniques used and summarizes studies addressing patients' outcomes using nerve blocks and their effect on postoperative cognition and function.

Conflicts: The authors have no conflicts of interest.

*Corresponding author. University of Pennsylvania, 3400 Spruce Street, Dulles 6, Philadelphia, PA 19104. *E-mail address*: Nabil.Elkassabany@uphs.upenn.edu

http://dx.doi.org/10.1016/j.aan.2016.07.007

BACKGROUND

Hip fractures are a common problem for older adults, both in the United States and across the world. There are an estimated 300,000 hip fractures each year in the United States and 1.6 million worldwide, with the number growing each year as the population ages and the prevalence of osteoporosis increases [1]. Hip fractures are associated with potentially devastating outcomes. At 1-year follow-up, 25% of hip fracture patients will have died, and 50% of patients who previously lived independently will die or require nursing home placement [2]. It is estimated that the cost of hip fractures among older adults in the United States is more than $5.4 billion annually [3,4].

The majority of hip fracture patients will require surgery. In a 2008 metaanalysis of 257,367 patients, a delay in surgery for greater than 48 hours after admission was associated with a 41% greater 30-day all-cause mortality, and a 32% higher 1-year all-cause mortality [5]. It is currently recommended that patients undergo surgery as soon as possible once they have been optimized medically [6].

Given the scope of the problem and the public health ramifications both in terms of morbidity and mortality and medical costs, better ways of treating patients with hip fractures are needed.

CHOICE OF ANESTHESIA AND OUTCOME

The most widely used options for the primary anesthetic modality during surgery include general anesthesia and central neuraxial (spinal or epidural) anesthesia. The question of whether neuraxial or general anesthesia provides superior patient outcomes after hip fractures remains to be definitively answered. Potential outcome benefits of neuraxial anesthesia techniques include avoidance of intubation and mechanical ventilation, decreased blood loss, better perioperative analgesia, less opioid use, and potentially less postoperative cognitive dysfunction (POCD) in this elderly population [6]. General anesthesia, in contrast, is thought to provide improved hemodynamic stability and thus may be potentially safer for patients. However, current studies have shown differing results and expert opinions are varied [7]. As a result, professional society guidelines are not able to definitively recommend 1 anesthetic technique over another, leading to a wide variation in anesthetic practice [8]. It has been hypothesized that this lack of standardization in practice may play a role in the persistently high rates of morbidity and mortality after hip fracture surgery [6]. The American Academy of Orthopedic Surgeons guidelines state that strong evidence supports similar outcomes for general or spinal anesthesia [8]. In 2011, the Guideline Development Group from the National Institute for Health and Care Excellence in the United Kingdom recommended that more studies are needed to answer the question as to the cost effectiveness of neuraxial versus general anesthesia on postoperative morbidity and mortality in patients with hip fracture, specifically randomized control trial designs [9].

Mortality

Whether spinal anesthesia for hip fracture surgery is associated with lower mortality is still debatable. The main reason resides in shortcomings of the study design and the heterogeneity in the results of different studies. Evidence is derived from either randomized clinical trials (RCTs) or retrospective cohort studies. Most of the RCTs designed to address the question of spinal versus general anesthesia are dated, from single institution (thus decreasing external validity), and smaller studies of less than 100 patients. At this point, these studies may not accurately reflect current clinical; practice, particularly with regard to contemporary general anesthetic techniques. A metaanalysis of the results of the RCTs was released initially published in 2004 and recently updated in 2016 [10] did not find a difference in short-term mortality at 30 days with a relative risk of 0.78 (95% confidence interval, 0.57–1.06) between general or central neuraxial anesthesia. In addition, there were no outcome differences for clinically relevant outcomes such as pneumonia, myocardial infarction, cerebrovascular accidents, or acute POCD. Another recently published systematic review also failed to demonstrate any outcome differences between general versus regional anesthesia.

In a pilot RCT of 322 patients with hip fracture, Parker and Griffiths [11] randomized patients to receive either general or spinal anesthesia. Interestingly, they found the 30-day mortality to be marginally better for patients who received spinal anesthesia, yet it was less for the general anesthesia group at the 1-year follow-up. The authors felt that the decrease in mortality at 1-year follow-up was likely to be a chance finding related to the small sample size because they found it difficult to explain how an effect from anesthetic technique that was not found at an earlier time point (30-day mortality) could affect outcomes at a later time point. Recently, Guay and colleagues [7] pooled the results of 28 RCTs with 2976 participants, comparing neuraxial with general anesthesia. They still did not find a difference for mortality at 1 month. The authors conclude that "large randomized trials reflecting actual clinical practice" are needed to draw definitive conclusions [7].

Retrospective cohort studies offer the advantage of looking at a large number of patients in readily available databases. However, these databases are not designed to collect clinical data and the data are retrospective in nature are limitations. Multiple statistical methods are used to adjust for the variables that may confound the association between the type of anesthesia and the outcome in question. A retrospective study of veterans with hip fracture showed that general anesthesia and delay of surgery more than 4 days from admission were associated with higher risk of 30-day mortality and in-hospital complications [12]. Neuman and colleagues [13] found a similar advantage for spinal over general anesthesia when they analyzed data from the New York State discharge database. Similarly, a propensity score-match analysis of a Taiwanese in-patient claims database showed that spinal anesthesia was associated with lower odds of death when compared with general anesthesia (odds ratio, 1.24; 95% confidence interval, 1.15–1.35) [14].

Other studies have shown no difference in mortality based on the anesthesia technique [15–20]. The study by Seitz and colleagues [18] compared 6135 matched pairs of older adults with dementia and found no differences in 30-day mortality. This study was unique in that it specifically studied patients with dementia, an important and likely increasing subgroup of the patient population with hip fracture.

Some authors [19] call into question whether mortality is the correct outcome to study when comparing spinal versus general anesthesia, because mortality at different points is influenced by multiple variables other than the anesthetic itself. Hence, it would be reasonable to recommend that further study focusing on finding the "best methods" of both spinal and general anesthesia for patients with hip fracture rather than attempting to definitively define one anesthesia type to be better than another. The definition of the potential "best methods" for further study can be optimizing perioperative pain control with local anesthetic nerve block; using lower doses of all anesthesia medications, whether for general or spinal anesthesia; and using no or very light sedation when administering spinal anesthesia.

Perioperative complications

Overall complications

There have been 3 recently published retrospective reviews of the large, multicenter American College of Surgeons' National Surgical Quality Improvement Program database. The first study compared operating room times, duration of stay, 30-day adverse events, and readmission rates for patients who had received either spinal or general anesthesia [21]. They found a higher likelihood of overall any adverse event, including a higher likelihood of thromboembolic events, minor adverse events, and blood transfusion, for patients undergoing general anesthesia. However, urinary tract infection was lower in the general anesthesia group. They also found general anesthesia to be associated with slightly longer operative time and postoperative time in the operating room, but did not find differences in postoperative duration of stay or readmission rates. In the second retrospective review, the authors found an increased risk for overall complications in patients receiving general anesthesia when compared with spinal anesthesia [22]. Similar to other recently published studies, they also did not find a difference in 30-day mortality between the 2 anesthesia types.

Conversely, the third study using the National Surgical Quality Improvement Program dataset found regional anesthesia to be associated with significantly higher likelihood of both minor and total number of perioperative complications in patients undergoing regional anesthesia when compared with patients undergoing general anesthesia [20]. In their analysis they found the odds of greater total complications from spinal anesthesia was driven mainly by greater odds of minor complications in the spinal anesthesia group, and this difference remained significant when patients who received regional nerve blocks were added to the spinal group. The authors acknowledge that their findings are at odds with the conclusions drawn from several prior studies and metaanalyses. They point out several perceived methodologic flaws in other studies that they feel may have contributed to these differences. Similarly, a 2011 systematic review included 83 studies on acute hip fracture [23] did not find evidence of significant differences in terms of preventing cardiac complications, deep venous thrombosis, and pulmonary embolism, although peripheral nerves blocks were shown to provide more effective perioperative analgesia compared with traditional systemic analgesics.

Perioperative stroke, respiratory failure, and admission to the intensive care unit were more frequent in patients receiving general anesthesia [14]. In this analysis, the general anesthesia group had a slightly longer hospital stay and higher costs of their hospitalization. Findings of this study suggested that hip fracture type and hospital characteristics may be associated with increased odds of postoperative complications and further research is needed to determine which patients would most benefit.

As mentioned, RCTs addressing the question of spinal versus general anesthesia were mostly single institution, had small sample size, and may not accurately reflect current practice, because some of the studies are old. Spinal anesthesia was associated with a lesser chance of deep venous thrombosis and less blood loss [10,24]. These findings may be scrutinized, because some of the studies included in the analysis predate the development of guidelines for prophylaxis against deep venous thrombosis.

In a pilot trial of 322 patients with hip fracture, Parker and Griffiths [11] randomized patients to receive either general anesthesia or spinal anesthesia. They did not find differences in outcome of hospital stay, need for blood transfusion or postoperative complications.

Pulmonary complications

There is also a potential for anesthesia type to affect outcomes in certain subsets of patient populations. In 1 retrospective study of veterans with hip fractures and chronic obstructive pulmonary disease, general anesthesia was identified as a modifiable risk factor with the potential that increased use of regional anesthesia could be used to improve patient outcomes in this particular patient population [25]. More studies are needed to identify other potential subgroups that may benefit from particular methods of anesthesia or analgesia.

A 2012 comparative effectiveness study of regional versus general anesthesia for hip fracture surgery found that the use of regional anesthesia was associated with a 29% decrease in mortality and a 24% decrease of inpatient pulmonary complications [13]. They did not find a difference with respect to cardiovascular complications. Interestingly, they found the benefit of regional anesthesia over general to hold true for intertrochanteric fractures, but not patients with femoral neck fractures. The authors call for futures studies to further explore which subsets of patients with hip fracture may benefit the most from certain anesthesia techniques.

Cognitive dysfunction and postoperative delirium

Spinal anesthesia has been suggested to have a protective effect against development of acute POCD and acute confusion state [10,24]. In contrast, a meta-analysis by Wu and colleagues [26] concluded that the use of intraoperative neuraxial anesthesia did not seem to decrease the incidence of POCD when compared with general anesthesia. The authors pointed to methodologic issues with each study design and to the different definition of POCD and different instruments used for its measurement. Similarly, other studies have come to the same conclusion [23].

The level of sedation used during regional anesthesia techniques for hip fracture surgery may influence the outcome in terms of postoperative delirium in this elderly patient population. Many of the studies on the topic of regional versus general anesthesia either do not control for or do not detail the level of sedation that was used during spinal anesthesia. One randomized controlled study looked at whether limiting intraoperative sedation during hip fracture repair would decrease the prevalence of delirium in the postoperative period [27]. In this trial, hip fracture repair was performed under spinal anesthesia with propofol sedation titrated using the bispectral index. The authors found the prevalence of postoperative delirium to be significantly lower in the light sedation group, with a number needed to treat of 4.7 patients to prevent 1 incident of delirium. The authors advocate for limiting intraoperative sedation as a simple and cost-effective method of improving patient care in this population.

Cost

A 2012 single-center retrospective study examined the effects of neuraxial anesthesia on morbidity, mortality, and hospitalization costs [28]. They did not find a difference in the rates of in-hospital mortality or rates of readmission. The average cost of hospitalization was $16,789. This number was not significantly different between the patients who received general or neuraxial anesthesia. However, delay before surgery and admission to an intensive care unit increased the cost of hospitalization.

In contrast, spinal anesthesia has been associated with lower hospital expenditure in the United Kingdom [29] and in Taiwan [14,30]. Although spinal anesthesia may seem to be financially preferable, it is difficult to draw conclusions as to the true monetary advantage of one versus the other because of the absence of definitive data on clinical outcome differences between the 2 anesthesia types. Chakladar and White [29] concluded that the time required to perform spinal anesthesia was approximately 4 minutes longer than the time needed for induction of general anesthesia. Although the total operating room time was not statistically different, possibly owing to the longer emergence time needed after general anesthesia.

PERIOPERATIVE PAIN MANAGEMENT

Pain management is an important component of care for patients both before and after hip fracture repair. Patients with high pain scores are found to be at greater risk for delirium, as well as having longer hospital stays [31,32]. They are less likely to mobilize after surgery and report poorer health-related quality of life [33,34]. Further complicating their care is the fact that many of these patients have cognitive impairment at baseline that may limit accurate assessment of their pain. The American Academy of Orthopedic Surgeons guidelines for management of hip fractures in the elderly finds "strong evidence supports regional analgesia to improve preoperative pain control in patients with hip fracture" [8].

A 2011 systematic review of pain management interventions for hip fracture included 83 studies investigating preoperative and intraoperative pain management for acute hip fracture [23]. Studies addressing the use nerve blockade found that the incidence of delirium was decreased when nerve blocks were used compared with no nerve block. No evidence was found to support one type of nerve block technique over another.

There are several options to provide pain relief postoperatively, including systemic analgesia with opioids and other adjuvant medications, and regional techniques such as femoral nerve block, fascia iliaca block, lumbar plexus block, and epidural analgesia. The potential outcome benefits of nerve blocks include superior analgesia, decreased use of opioids in this elderly population, and possible decreases in rates of postoperative delirium or POCD [35]. Patients with hip fractures are usually in severe pain at presentation to the emergency department. The hip joint is innervated by a combination of branches from the femoral, obturator, superior gluteal, sciatic nerve, and nerve to the quadratus femoris. Therefore, no single peripheral injection site is able to provide sufficient coverage [36].

Fascia iliaca and femoral nerve block for preoperative and postoperative analgesia

Several studies have looked at the possibilities to improve postoperative pain management as well as the effect on other patient outcomes with fascia iliaca or femoral nerve block. The effects of fascia iliaca compartment block are thought to come from spread of local anesthetic under the fascia iliaca to block the femoral, lateral femoral cutaneous, and obturator nerves [37].

The American Academy of Orthopedic Surgeons recommendation was based on analysis of the results of 6 RCTs [38–43] that involved a total of 593 patients. All studies found a decrease in preoperative pain after either a fascia iliaca compartment block or a femoral nerve block. In 1 study, fascia iliaca block was found to not only decrease preoperative pain, but also to have effects beyond the preoperative period with a decreased incidence of delirium postoperatively [42]. In a small study of 68 patients, placing a preoperative epidural in patients with cardiac disease was associated with decreased preoperative adverse cardiac events [44]. However, the incidence of intraoperative and postoperative cardiac events was similar between the 2 groups.

Few studies have looked at the potential for fascia iliaca compartment block or femoral nerve block to be performed immediately on presentation to the emergency department with the goal to decrease the initial use of systemic opioids. In a double-blind, placebo-controlled study of 48 patients randomized to either fascia iliaca block with local anesthetic and placebo intramuscular saline or placebo fascia iliaca block with saline and intramuscular injection of morphine pain control was found to be better at all measured time points in the true fascia iliaca block group [38]. However, patients were only followed until 180 minutes after the block had been performed.

In another study, fascia iliaca block was used preoperatively to help improve pain control during patient positioning for spinal anesthesia [45]. They found that performing fascia iliaca block 20 minutes before positioning for spinal anesthesia was associated with lower pain scores at all measured time points, shorter time of spinal performance and better quality of positioning, lower use of morphine postoperatively and increased patient satisfaction rates when compared with use of intravenous fentanyl injection. Thus, preoperative nerve block was likely to improve both the quality and the efficiency of care for these patients.

Additional regional anesthetic techniques

A recent multiple treatment comparison review was used to look at whether there is evidence to recommend a particular nerve block technique for perioperative pain control for patients with hip fracture [35]. In this study, the authors found the combination of obturator and lateral femoral cutaneous nerve blocks most likely to be effective for acute postoperative pain control and fascia iliaca block most likely to lead to reduced rates of postoperative delirium. They did not find a significant difference in terms of the other regional techniques studied including epidural analgesia, femoral nerve block, psoas compartment block, "3 in 1" technique, or lumbar sacral plexus block. It is hypothesized that fascia iliaca block may offer potential benefits with limited risks over femoral nerve block in the acute setting because the site of injection is further away from nerves or blood vessels. The authors further postulate that blocking the lateral femoral cutaneous nerve of the thigh plays an important role in treating the pain from soft tissue disruption that occurs as part of the surgical approach to hip fracture repair; and perhaps this is in part why patients who received fascia iliaca nerve block and the combination of obturator/lateral femoral cutaneous nerve performed the best.

FUTURE DIRECTIONS

There are more recent data that regional anesthesia and analgesia may be associated with improved outcomes (such as improved analgesia and decreased site infection–associated readmission) in patients undergoing surgery for hip fracture repair [46,47]. This effect needs to be elucidated in prospective multicenter RCTs that will encompass the variability of clinical practice between different institutions. The other question that needs to be addressed is which outcomes should we be looking at? We believe that we should be looking at other clinically important outcomes, which are most important from the patient perspective. Functional outcomes and return to normal daily routine are a few to be named.

SUMMARY

There seems to be a role for regional anesthesia and analgesia on improving outcomes for patients with hip fractures, although this role has not been completely defined yet. More studies are needed to better identify which anesthetic techniques are most beneficial, and perhaps which subsets of patients will benefit from particular regional techniques mostly.

References

[1] Brauer CA, Coca-Perraillon M, Cutler DM, et al. Incidence and mortality of hip fractures in the United States. JAMA 2009;302(14):1573–9.

[2] Tajeu GS, Delzell E, Smith W, et al. Death, debility, and destitution following hip fracture. J Gerontol A Biol Sci Med Sci 2014;69(3):346–53.

[3] Roudsari BS, Ebel BE, Corso PS, et al. The acute medical care costs of fall-related injuries among the U.S. older adults. Injury 2005;36(11):1316–22.

[4] Braithwaite RS, Col NF, Wong JB. Estimating hip fracture morbidity, mortality and costs. J Am Geriatr Soc 2003;51(3):364–70.

[5] Shiga T, Wajima Z, Ohe Y. Is operative delay associated with increased mortality of hip fracture patients? Systematic review, meta-analysis, and meta-regression. Can J Anaesth 2008;55(3):146–54.

[6] Mears SC, Kates SL. A guide to improving the care of patients with fragility fractures, edition 2. Geriatr Orthop Surg Rehabil 2015;6(2):58–120.

[7] Guay J, Parker MJ, Gajendragadkar PR, et al. Anaesthesia for hip fracture surgery in adults. Cochrane Database Syst Rev 2016;(2):CD000521.

[8] Roberts KC, Brox WT. AAOS clinical practice guideline: management of hip fractures in the elderly. J Am Acad Orthop Surg 2015;23(2):138–40.

[9] The management of hip fracture in adults. London (United Kingdom): National Clinical Guideline Center, Royal College of Physicians; 2011.

[10] Parker MJ, Handoll HH, Griffiths R. Anaesthesia for hip fracture surgery in adults. Cochrane Database Syst Rev 2016;(2):CD000521.

[11] Parker MJ, Griffiths R. General versus regional anaesthesia for hip fractures. A pilot randomised controlled trial of 322 patients. Injury 2015;46(8):1562–6.

[12] Radcliff TA, Henderson WG, Stoner TJ, et al. Patient risk factors, operative care, and outcomes among older community-dwelling male veterans with hip fracture. J Bone Joint Surg Am 2008;90(1):34–42.

[13] Neuman MD, Silber JH, Elkassabany NM, et al. Comparative effectiveness of regional versus general anesthesia for hip fracture surgery in adults. Anesthesiology 2012;117(1):72–92.

[14] Chu CC, Weng SF, Chen KT, et al. Propensity score-matched comparison of postoperative adverse outcomes between geriatric patients given a general or a neuraxial anesthetic for hip surgery: a population-based study. Anesthesiology 2015;123(1):136–47.

[15] Neuman MD, Rosenbaum PR, Ludwig JM, et al. Anesthesia technique, mortality, and length of stay after hip fracture surgery. JAMA 2014;311(24):2508–17.

[16] O'Hara DA, Duff A, Berlin JA, et al. The effect of anesthetic technique on postoperative outcomes in hip fracture repair. Anesthesiology 2000;92(4):947–57.

[17] Patorno E, Neuman MD, Schneeweiss S, et al. Comparative safety of anesthetic type for hip fracture surgery in adults: retrospective cohort study. BMJ 2014;348:g4022.

[18] Seitz DP, Anderson GM, Austin PC, et al. Effects of impairment in activities of daily living on predicting mortality following hip fracture surgery in studies using administrative healthcare databases. BMC Geriatr 2014;14:9.

[19] White SM, Moppett IK, Griffiths R. Outcome by mode of anaesthesia for hip fracture surgery. An observational audit of 65 535 patients in a national dataset. Anaesthesia 2014;69(3):224–30.

[20] Whiting PS, Molina CS, Greenberg SE, et al. Regional anaesthesia for hip fracture surgery is associated with significantly more peri-operative complications compared with general anaesthesia. Int Orthop 2015;39(7):1321–7.
[21] Basques BA, Bohl DD, Golinvaux NS, et al. General versus spinal anaesthesia for patients aged 70 years and older with a fracture of the hip. Bone Joint J 2015;97-B(5):689–95.
[22] Fields AC, Dieterich JD, Buterbaugh K, et al. Short-term complications in hip fracture surgery using spinal versus general anaesthesia. Injury 2015;46(4):719–23.
[23] Abou-Setta AM, Beaupre LA, Rashiq S, et al. Comparative effectiveness of pain management interventions for hip fracture: a systematic review. Ann Intern Med 2011;155(4): 234–45.
[24] Oliver D, Griffiths R, Roche J, et al. Hip fracture. BMJ Clin Evid 2010;2010.
[25] Maciejewski ML, Radcliff TA, Henderson WG, et al. Determinants of postsurgical discharge setting for male hip fracture patients. J Rehabil Res Dev 2013;50(9):1267–76.
[26] Wu CL, Hsu W, Richman JM, et al. Postoperative cognitive function as an outcome of regional anesthesia and analgesia. Reg Anesth Pain Med 2004;29(3):257–68.
[27] Sieber FE, Zakriya KJ, Gottschalk A, et al. Sedation depth during spinal anesthesia and the development of postoperative delirium in elderly patients undergoing hip fracture repair. Mayo Clin Proc 2010;85(1):18–26.
[28] Le-Wendling L, Bihorac A, Baslanti TO, et al. Regional anesthesia as compared with general anesthesia for surgery in geriatric patients with hip fracture: does it decrease morbidity, mortality, and health care costs? Results of a single-centered study. Pain Med 2012;13(7): 948–56.
[29] Chakladar A, White SM. Cost estimates of spinal versus general anaesthesia for fractured neck of femur surgery. Anaesthesia 2010;65(8):810–4.
[30] White SM, Sanghera P, Chakladar A. Leukocytosis increases length of inpatient stay but not age-adjusted 30-day mortality, after hip fracture. Age Ageing 2010;39(5):650–3.
[31] Morrison RS, Magaziner J, McLaughlin MA, et al. The impact of post-operative pain on outcomes following hip fracture. Pain 2003;103(3):303–11.
[32] Morrison RS, Magaziner J, Gilbert M, et al. Relationship between pain and opioid analgesics on the development of delirium following hip fracture. J Gerontol A Biol Sci Med 2003;58(1):76–81.
[33] Van Balen R, Essink-Bot ML, Steyerberg E, et al. Quality of life after hip fracture: a comparison of four health status measures in 208 patients. Disabil Rehabil 2003;25(10):507–19.
[34] Herrick C, Steger-May K, Sinacore DR, et al. Persistent pain in frail older adults after hip fracture repair. J Am Geriatr Soc 2004;52(12):2062–8.
[35] Rashiq S, Vandermeer B, Abou-Setta AM, et al. Efficacy of supplemental peripheral nerve blockade for hip fracture surgery: multiple treatment comparison. Can J Anaesth 2013;60(3):230–43.
[36] Birnbaum K, Prescher A, Hessler S, et al. The sensory innervation of the hip joint–an anatomical study. Surg Radiol Anat 1997;19(6):371–5.
[37] Capdevila X, Biboulet P, Bouregba M, et al. Comparison of the three-in-one and fascia iliaca compartment blocks in adults: clinical and radiographic analysis. Anesth Analg 1998;86(5):1039–44.
[38] Foss NB, Kristensen BB, Bundgaard M, et al. Fascia iliaca compartment blockade for acute pain control in hip fracture patients: a randomized, placebo-controlled trial. Anesthesiology 2007;106(4):773–8.
[39] Fletcher AK, Rigby AS, Heyes FL. Three-in-one femoral nerve block as analgesia for fractured neck of femur in the emergency department: a randomized, controlled trial. Ann Emerg Med 2003;41(2):227–33.
[40] Haddad FS, Williams RL. Femoral nerve block in extracapsular femoral neck fractures. J Bone Joint Surg Br 1995;77(6):922–3.

[41] Godoy Monzon D, Vazquez J, Jauregui JR, et al. Pain treatment in post-traumatic hip fracture in the elderly: regional block vs. systemic non-steroidal analgesics. Int J Emerg Med 2010;3(4):321–5.
[42] Mouzopoulos G, Vasiliadis G, Lasanianos N, et al. Fascia iliaca block prophylaxis for hip fracture patients at risk for delirium: a randomized placebo-controlled study. J Orthop Traumatol 2009;10(3):127–33.
[43] Yun MJ, Kim YH, Han MK, et al. Analgesia before a spinal block for femoral neck fracture: fascia iliaca compartment block. Acta Anaesthesiol Scand 2009;53(10):1282–7.
[44] Matot I, Oppenheim-Eden A, Ratrot R, et al. Preoperative cardiac events in elderly patients with hip fracture randomized to epidural or conventional analgesia. Anesthesiology 2003;98(1):156–63.
[45] Diakomi M, Papaioannou M, Mela A, et al. Preoperative fascia iliaca compartment block for positioning patients with hip fractures for central nervous blockade: a randomized trial. Reg Anesth Pain Med 2014;39(5):394–8.
[46] Ritcey B, Pageau P, Woo MY, et al. Regional nerve blocks for hip and femoral neck fractures in the emergency department: a systematic review. CJEM 2016;18:37–47.
[47] Tung YC, Hsu YH, Chang GM. The effect of anesthetic type on outcomes of hip fracture surgery: a nationwide population-based study. Medicine (Baltimore) 2016;95:e3296.

Advances in Anesthesia 34 (2016) 117–141

ADVANCES IN ANESTHESIA

ELSEVIER
MOSBY

The Perioperative Management of Implantable Pacemakers and Cardioverter-Defibrillators

Peter M. Schulman, MD[a,*], Marc A. Rozner, PhD, MD[b,c]

[a]Department of Anesthesiology and Perioperative Medicine, Oregon Health & Science University, Mail Code KPV 5A, 3181 Southwest Sam Jackson Park Road, Portland, OR 97239, USA; [b]Department of Anesthesiology and Perioperative Medicine, The University of Texas MD Anderson Cancer Center, 1400 Holcombe Boulevard, Unit Number: 0409, Houston, TX 77030, USA; [c]Department of Cardiology, The University of Texas MD Anderson Cancer Center, Houston, TX, USA

Keywords

- Pacemaker • Implantable cardioverter-defibrillator
- Cardiovascular implantable electronic device (CIED)
- Electromagnetic interference

Key points

- In addition to delivering high-voltage therapy, all modern transvenous implantable cardioverter-defibrillators (ICDs) can also perform all the sophisticated, advanced functions of a pacemaker (PM) (ie, all ICDs also have anti-bradyarrhythmia capability).
- Before elective surgery, ensuring that the patient's cardiovascular implantable electronic device (CIED) is functioning properly remains paramount, especially for surgery that is likely to result in hemodynamic embarrassment or whenever electromagnetic interference (ie, the use of monopolar electrosurgery) is likely. In any situation wherein a preoperative device evaluation cannot take place (ie, emergency surgery), practitioners must be prepared for perioperative device malfunction or outright failure. This preparation often includes the placement of transcutaneous pacing/defibrillation pads.

Continued

*Corresponding author. *E-mail address:* schulman@ohsu.edu

http://dx.doi.org/10.1016/j.aan.2016.07.008

Continued

- Electrical instruments, principally monopolar electrosurgery, but also those used by anesthesiologists (eg, nerve stimulators, radiofrequency scanning devices), can create electromagnetic interference and adversely affect the function of a CIED. If intra-operative electromagnetic interference is anticipated, ICD high-voltage therapy (anti-tachycardia pacing and shock) should be disabled and external defibrillation pads applied. Reprogramming to an asynchronous pacing mode should also be considered for any pacing-dependent patient.
- Except under exigent circumstances, magnet behavior should be confirmed whenever magnet use is planned. A magnet never alters the pacing mode of an ICD. It is sometimes possible to disable a CIED's magnet response through programming. Especially for an ICD, it might be difficult to determine that a CIED's magnet mode is disabled.
- Perioperative practitioners must be alert to incorrectly displayed electrocardiographic signals and rates resulting from electromagnetic interference.

INTRODUCTION: NATURE OF THE PROBLEM

In the United States, more than 3 million people have an implantable pacemaker (PM) or cardioverter-defibrillator (ICD) [1], and more than 500,000 PMs and ICDs are now implanted each year [2–5]. Initially developed to manage symptomatic bradyarrhythmias and sustained ventricular tachyarrhythmias, these cardiovascular implantable electronic devices (CIEDs) and their indications for use have evolved considerably, including treatment for heart failure [6]. Moreover, patients receiving these devices are older and have increasing medical comorbidities [3]. Although the incidence of patients with a CIED undergoing surgery is currently unknown, this number is likely substantial because these devices are so prevalent and more than 80 million surgical procedures are performed annually in the United States [7,8]. Also, some published reports suggest that the number of potentially eligible patients not receiving ICD therapy is sizable, but that a higher proportion of eligible patients might receive devices going forward [9,10]. Consequently, clinicians involved in perioperative care should expect to encounter and manage these patients with increasing frequency. Thus, anesthesiologists, just like general cardiologists, must become proficient in certain basic aspects of CIED therapy [6].

Unfortunately, the broad functionality of modern CIEDs has increased their complexity. As a result, safe, efficient, and cost-effective perioperative care of patients with CIED has become confounded by economic, personnel, and procedural challenges. The sophistication of these devices, the abundance of complex issues surrounding effective perioperative management of the patient with CIED, and changing patient conditions has increased the difficulty of providing this care. At least 2 reports suggest an association between these devices and increased perioperative morbidity and mortality [11,12]. Particular challenges include manufacturer-specific proprietary features, lack of standardization among device manufacturers, and an array of published literature that is often outdated and sometimes incorrect. Furthermore, in the operating or procedure room, electrical equipment emitting virtually uncontrolled radiofrequency signals (especially monopolar electrosurgical devices) can affect CIED function and place patients at increased risk of adverse events. Moreover, the presence of a CIED complicates operative scheduling and might introduce operative delays [13].

In response to these challenges, the Heart Rhythm Society (HRS) [14], American Society of Anesthesiologists (ASA) [15], and others [16,17] have published recommendations to guide clinicians in the perioperative management of patients with these devices. These recommendations delineate that, preoperatively, these patients must be identified before arrival at the surgical facility, because proper CIED function must be verified and a comprehensive plan ("perioperative prescription") for managing the CIED must be established that accounts for the patient, the anticipated procedure, and the individual characteristics of the patient's CIED [18]. Although in many instances this management plan can be created by accessing the patient's records and without performing a de novo device interrogation, CIED records sometimes are not readily available to the operative care team on the day of the procedure. In addition, even when a de novo device interrogation is not required, immediate preoperative reprogramming might be needed to mitigate the risks of electromagnetic interference (EMI) arising from the use of radiofrequency instruments, primarily monopolar electrosurgery (electrosurgical unit [ESU]). Although allied health professionals such as manufacturer representatives are frequently engaged to prescribe or independently deliver such care, this practice should be avoided [14]. Moreover, appropriately trained, licensed, and privileged practitioners (typically cardiologists or specially trained advance practice providers) are often not available and are not well incentivized to perform this service on a timely basis, particularly if they do not routinely provide perioperative care. In this situation, routine placement of a magnet over a CIED, presumably to change the pacing mode of a PM or suspend the antitachycardia therapies of an ICD, has been used. However, blind application of a magnet to a CIED during surgery can lead to adverse outcomes [19] and is no longer considered acceptable except under exigent circumstances [14].

Although anesthesiologists and surgeons are not expected to become CIED management experts, any practitioner involved in the perioperative care of patients with CIED should be familiar with the key published practice recommendations and expert consensus statements on this topic. Furthermore, they should understand indications for CIED implantation, along with the basic functions, operations, and limitations of these devices. Finally, they should have enough troubleshooting knowledge to know when expert consultation is warranted.

This review provides the perioperative clinician with a comprehensive understanding of the considerations involved in the safe and effective perioperative management of the patient with a CIED.

The perioperative management of the patient with CIED can be divided into 3 distinct periods: preoperative, intraoperative, and postoperative.

PREOPERATIVE EVALUATION AND MANAGEMENT

Preoperatively, information about the CIED system, patient, and procedure must be obtained (Box 1). The CIED team, anesthesiologist, and proceduralist should review this information and create an appropriate perioperative CIED management plan (see Box 1).

The cardiovascular implantable electronic devices system

CIED systems classically consist of a pulse generator and 1 to 3 leads (Fig. 1). The pulse generator is typically implanted underneath the clavicle (most often on the left side) in a subcutaneous pectoral pocket and the leads are almost always routed directly into the endocardium (heart) transvenously via the superior vena cava. Transvenous leads pace and sense in their respective locations and may be placed into the right atrium, right ventricle (RV), or coronary sinus (CS). The number of leads inserted is determined by the indications for implantation and specific CIED functionality required. An atrial lead is placed for sinus node dysfunction as well as atrial monitoring. RV leads can be used to circumvent atrioventricular (AV) block as well as monitor RV rhythm. Patients in the United States with sinoatrial node disease but without AV block at the time of implant generally still receive an RV lead because of the concern that AV block might develop later [20]. A CS lead is used to pace the left ventricle for cardiac resynchronization therapy (CRT); the position of the CS lead is best determined by lateral (rather than pulmonary artery) chest radiograph (CXR) (Fig. 2). The RV lead of a transvenous ICD contains 1 or 2 shock coils for high-voltage defibrillation therapy. The presence of shock coils can be used to easily distinguish a high-voltage capable device (ICD) from a PM via CXR (Fig. 3), although an ICD's high-voltage therapy might be programmed off at any given time. Of note, in addition to delivering anti-tachyarrhythmia therapy (including anti-tachycardia pacing [ATP] and shocks), all modern transvenous ICDs can perform all the sophisticated functions of a PM (ie, also have anti-bradyarrhythmia capability).

Transvenous leads can be either unipolar or bipolar. With a bipolar lead, the cathode and anode are both present on the lead itself (near the distal end), whereas with a unipolar lead, the cathode is present on the lead and the pulse generator functions as the anode (Fig. 4). Thus, the distance between the cathode and anode is decreased with a bipolar lead, reducing susceptibility to EMI during sensing. PMs (but usually not ICDs) with bipolar leads can be programmed to the unipolar mode for pacing and/or sensing. Sometimes, a PM automatically switches from a bipolar to unipolar pacing and sensing configuration if a lead fault is detected.

Newer CIED systems include a subcutaneous ICD (S-ICD) and leadless PM. The S-ICD (Fig. 5), which gained US Food and Drug Administration (FDA) approval in 2012, has 2 main components, a pulse generator and subcutaneously tunneled single-coil electrode that allows the device to sense malignant cardiac rhythms and deliver a shock when indicted. Because the electrode is implanted under the skin rather than in the heart, the potential for both acute

Box 1: Perioperative evaluation and management

Perioperative evaluation and management

1. CIED system
   a. Identify the presence of a CIED
   b. Determine (a) the CIED type (ie, PM, ICD, CRT), (b) generator manufacturer, (c) indication for implantation, (d) battery status, (e) current programming (including magnet response)
   c. Ensure proper CIED function, especially for surgery that is likely to result in hemodynamic embarrassment or whenever EMI (ie, which most commonly stems from the use of monopolar electrosurgery) is likely. (Proper function may often be established by querying the patient's medical record to determine when the CIED was last interrogated, and by accessing that interrogation report. CIEDs should be evaluated every 3–12 months, with shorter intervals recommended for patients with more complicated devices [ie, CRT systems] or medical conditions, or devices under alert notification).
2. Patient
   a. Determine the patient's underlying rate and rhythm, and whether the patient is pacing dependent.
   b. Evaluate the patient for and optimize coexisting disease or diseases.

Procedure

1. Determine whether intraoperative EMI is anticipated
2. If EMI is anticipated, (a) disable antitachycardia therapy if an ICD; (b) consider asynchronous pacing for the pacing-dependent patient.

(Note: Magnet application might be acceptable for some PMs (provide asynchronous pacing) or ICDs [disable antitachycardia therapy]. Asynchronous pacing from an ICD requires reprogramming.)

3. Consider additional programming changes, including
   a. Increasing the lower rate limit (ie, pacing rate) to optimize oxygen delivery (especially for major surgery)
   b. Programming to off (when present) pacing features that can mimic pacing system malfunction. These features include
      i. Minute ventilation rate response
      ii. Sleep rate (note that CIED clocks will not automatically adjust for travel or daylight savings time)
      iii. Hysteresis rate (pacing onset can be delayed by an intrinsic event)
      iv. Rate drop (high rate pacing, typically 100 bpm after a sudden drop in intrinsic rate is observed, which can be triggered by EMI)
      v. Right ventricular pacing avoidance algorithms that might
         1. Allow prolonged AV delay (to 450 milliseconds)
            a. Biotronik Vp suppression mode
            b. St Jude Medical ventricular intrinsic preference

2. Allow dropped QRS events
    a. Boston Scientific RYTHMIQ
    b. Medtronic managed ventricular pacing
    c. Sorin AAI-SafeR

Intraoperative management

1. Monitor cardiac rhythm/peripheral pulse with pulse oximeter plethysmogram or arterial waveform
2. Disable the artifact filter on the ECG monitor, although some advisories offer caution when doing so, because the painting of noncapturing artifacts might confuse perioperative personnel
3. Whenever feasible, avoid use of monopolar electrosurgery (ESU)
4. Position the ESU dispersive electrode to divert electricity away from the generator-heart circuit, even if the pad must be placed on the distal forearm and the wire covered with sterile drape
5. If the ESU causes ventricular oversensing, pacing quiescence, or inappropriate tachycardia, limit the effect by suspending the use of monopolar electrocautery, reprogramming the cardiac generator, or placing a magnet over the PM (not indicated for ICD)

Postoperative management

1. Any CIED that underwent preoperative or intraoperative reprogramming should be reinterrogated and have its parameters restored or optimized for perioperative recovery. Postoperative CIED interrogation should always be prompted by intraoperative hemodynamic instability or any concern for inappropriate CIED function.
2. The ICD patient must remain in a fully monitored setting (postanesthesia care unit or intensive care unit) until antitachycardia therapy is restored.

Adapted from Crossley GH, Poole JE, Rozner MA, et al. The Heart Rhythm Society (HRS)/American Society of Anesthesiologists (ASA) Expert Consensus Statement on the Perioperative Management of Patients with Implantable Defibrillators, Pacemakers and Arrhythmia Monitors: Facilities and Patient Management this document was developed as a joint project with the American Society of Anesthesiologists (ASA), and in collaboration with the American Heart Association (AHA), and the Society of Thoracic Surgeons (STS). Heart Rhythm 2011;8:1114–54.

(ie, pneumothorax, lead dislodgement, perforation, and endocarditis) and long-term (ie, lead failure, infection) complications are reduced or entirely avoided. The downside of this option is limited functionality; the high-voltage output is fixed at 80 J (ie, is nonprogrammable), and the system does not provide sophisticated antitachycardia or antibradycardia pacing nor can it offer treatment for heart failure (ie, CRT). It may also not be the best option for patients with recurrent monomorphic ventricular tachycardia (VT) because this rhythm can often be terminated with ATP, a feature that is available in all transvenous ICDs but which is not available in current S-ICD models [21]. Another emerging technology is the Leadless PM (Fig. 6), which provides

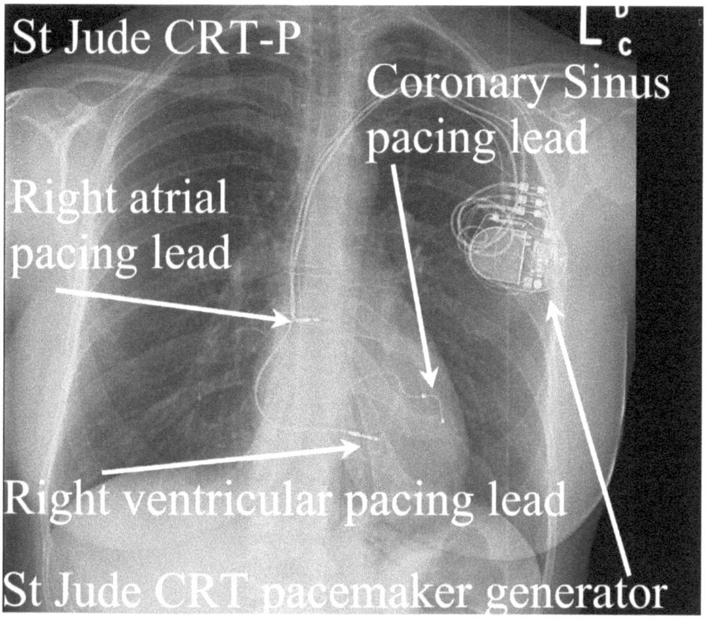

Fig. 1. A cardiac resynchronization pacemaker (CRT-P). The presence of a lead in the CS vein typically identifies a system as CRT. The absence of any shock coil defines this system as CRT-P (as opposed to CRT-D, which would be a cardiac resynchronization system with defibrillation capability).

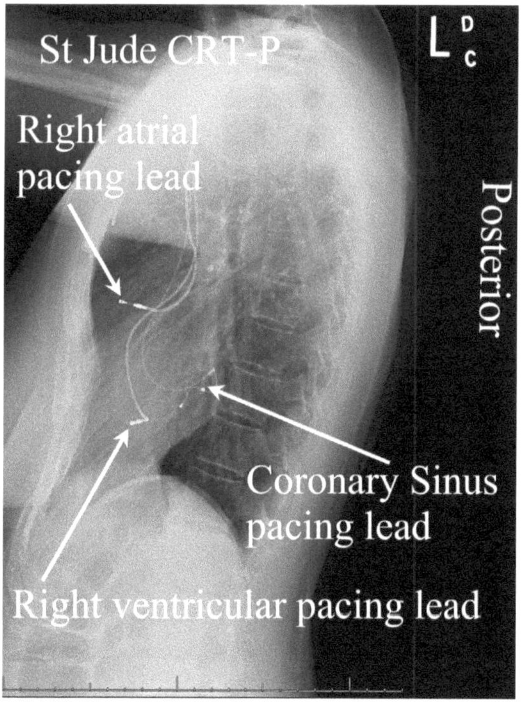

Fig. 2. A lateral CXR demonstrating the posterior position of the CS lead.

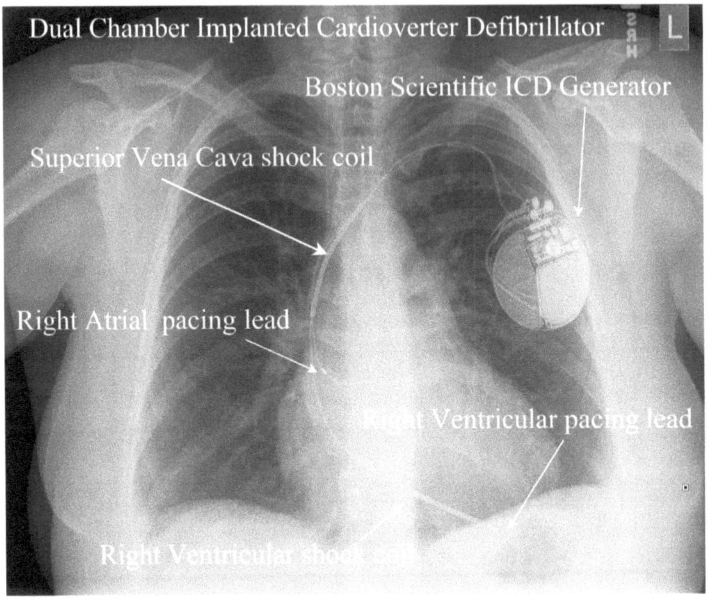

Fig. 3. A dual-chamber ICD system is shown. The presence of a shock coil in the RV (this device has an additional shock coil in the superior vena cava) identifies this CIED as a high-energy capable system, although without knowledge of the actual programming high-energy delivery cannot be assured. In most patients, the presence of an additional shock coil in the superior vena cava lowers the defibrillation threshold.

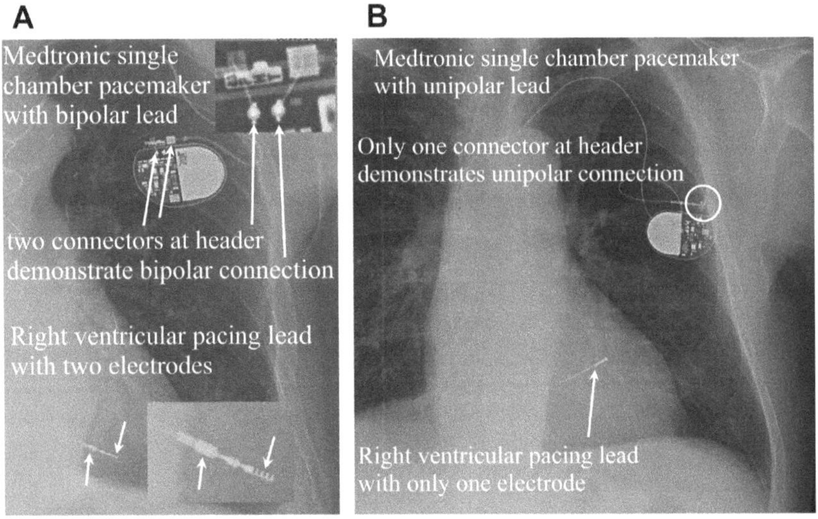

Fig. 4. (*A*) A single-chamber PM with a dedicated unipolar pacing/sensing lead is shown. The radiograph depiction clearly shows only one connector at the generator header. In a unipolar system, the generator always serves as the anode. (*B*) A single-chamber PM with a dedicated bipolar pacing/sensing lead is shown. For the lead in the RV, the downward arrow points to the cathode at the lead tip (which in this case is an active fixation screw). The upward arrow identifies the ring or anode electrode. At the top of the figure, 2 connectors can be seen at the generator header. Note that any bipolar lead can also be configured in unipolar mode, and for some advanced and newer generators, the selection of lead tip or ring as cathode is programmable.

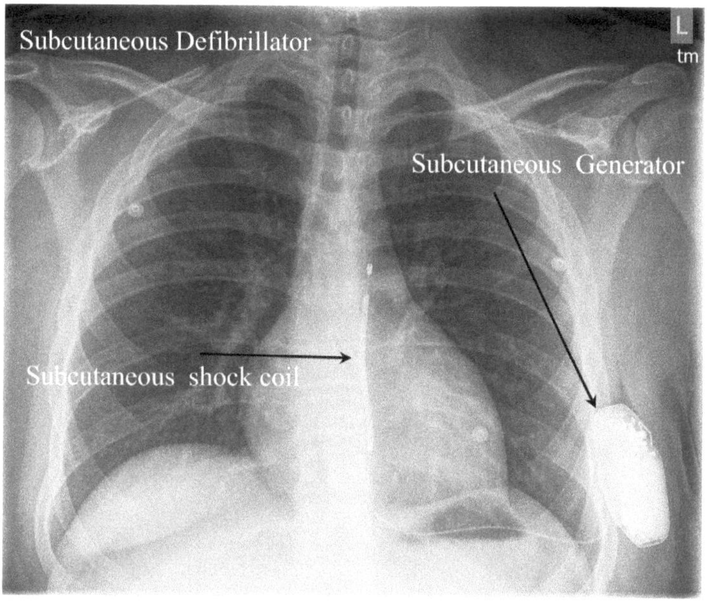

Fig. 5. A subcutaneous ICD (Boston Scientific, Marlborough, MA) is shown. In this case, the lead was tunneled at the level of the diaphragm. The longitudinal position of the shock coil is typical. The S-ICD has no ATP and very limited antibradycardia pacing (it paces for approximately 30 seconds after delivering a shock).

single-chamber RV pacing, is about one-tenth the size of a traditional PM, and is implanted through a catheter. Two versions (Nanostim [St. Jude Medical, Syl Mar, CA] and Micra [Medtronic Inc, Minneapolis, MN]) have a CE mark, and one (Medtronic Micra) has received FDA approval (April, 2016) and will thus become widely available in the United States in the near future. Perioperative clinicians who depend on magnet application to a CIED in the setting of EMI must understand that the magnet behavior of both the S-ICD and the Leadless PM is different from their traditional counterparts (see later discussion on magnet behavior).

A third minimally invasive nontherapeutic CIED is the implantable loop recorder (Fig. 7), a subcutaneous single-lead electrocardiogram (ECG) monitoring device used for diagnostic purposes only.

Understanding CIED nomenclature is necessary when caring for patients with these devices. The Pacemaking Code of the North American Society of Pacing and Electrophysiology and the British Pacing and Electrophysiology Group (NBG) provides a generic understanding of the antibradycardia programming of any CIED [22] (Table 1). The code has 5 positions: position I describes the chamber(s) paced; position II describes the chamber(s) sensed; position III describes how the CIED responds to a sensed event; position IV uses an "R" to denote the presence of rate modulation; and position V

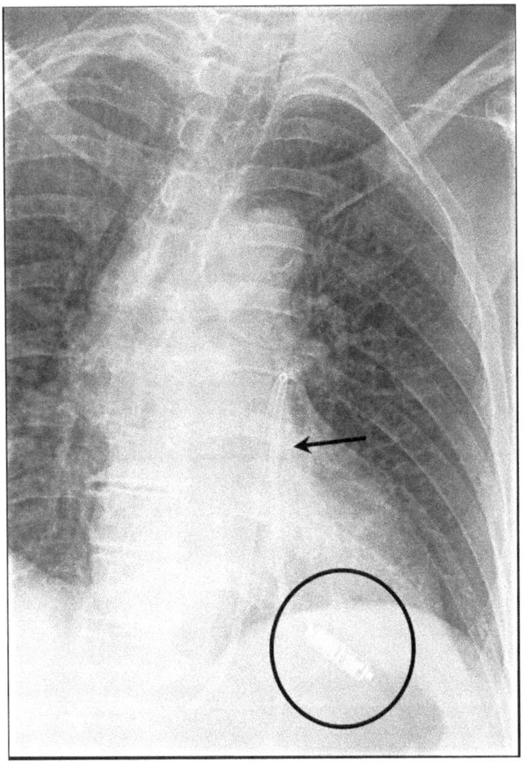

Fig. 6. A leadless PM (Medtronic) is shown (*circle*). The development of a pericardial effusion during PM implantation necessitated insertion of a pericardial drain (*arrow*). As noted in the text, currently all leadless PMs pace only in the VVI mode; thus they cannot provide AV synchrony or optimal hemodynamics. The Medtronic leadless PM has no magnet response. The St Jude leadless PM (not shown) responds to magnet placement with asynchronous (VOO) pacing, although not at constant rate (see text).

describes the presence or absence of multisite pacing (ie, biventricular pacing or CRT). Although not used as often as the NBG Code, transvenous ICDs have a 4-place generic NBD code [23] (Table 2) to indicate lead placement and device function. Position I indicates the chamber(s) shocked; position II indicates the chamber(s) in which ATP is administered; position III identifies the detection method (electrogram signals or hemodynamic sensor; not currently available in the United States); and position IV indicates the chamber(s) delivering antibradycardia pacing [22]. (Many PMs and ICDs now have antiatrial tachycardia, which includes ATP and low-energy cardioversion.) Because all transvenous ICDs can perform pacing for bradycardia, the most comprehensive description includes the first 3 characters of the NBD, followed by a dash, then the 5-character PM NBG [24].

Although traditional CIED systems are generally extremely reliable, system malfunction is not as rare as might be expected [25], and unfortunately, the first

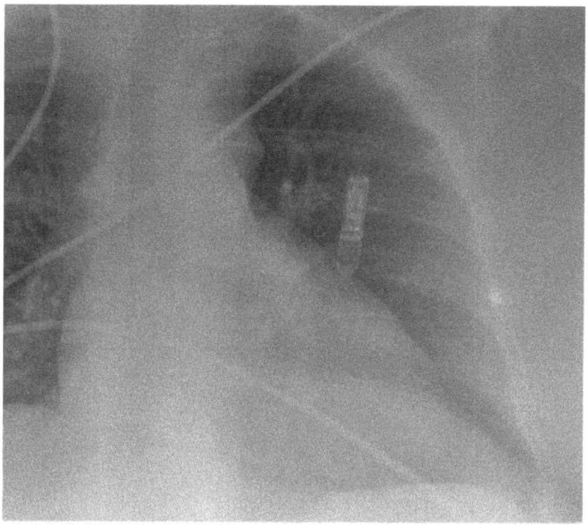

Fig. 7. An implanted loop recorder (in this case, a Medtronic LINQ) is shown in a typical subcutaneous implant position. Note the absence of leads.

indication of system failure can be death [26]. Maisel and colleagues [27] evaluated an FDA database to determine the general failure rate of these devices and found that over the 12-year study period (1990–2002), per 1000 implants, 4.6 PMs and 20.7 ICDs were explanted for issues other than battery depletion. During this time, 2.25 million PMs and 415,780 ICDs were implanted, and 30 PM and 31 ICD patients died as a direct result of device malfunction. In a subsequent analysis, Laskey and colleagues [28] reviewed FDA records from 2003 to 2007 for transvenous ICD explantations (459,000 transvenous ICDs and 256,000 CRT-Ds) and found 10,593 (2.3%) transvenous-ICD and 1925 (0.8%) CRT-D failures.

Table 1
The revised North American Society for Pacing and Electrophysiology/British Pacing and Electrophysiology Group generic code for antibradycardia, adaptive rate, and multisite pacing

Position I	Position II	Position III	Position IV	Position V
Pacing Chamber(s)	Sensing Chamber(s)	Response(s) to Sensing	Programmability	Multisite Pacing
O = None	*O* = None	*O* = None	*O* = None	*O* = None
A = Atrium	*A* = Atrium	*I* = Inhibited	*R* = Rate modulation	*A* = Atrium
V = Ventricle	*V* = Ventricle	*T* = Triggered		*V* = Ventricle
D = Dual (A + V)	*D* = Dual (A + V)	*D* = Dual (T + I)		*D* = Dual (A + V)

Adapted from Bernstein AD, Daubert JC, Fletcher RD, et al. The revised NASPE/BPEG generic code for antibradycardia, adaptive-rate, and multisite pacing. North American Society of Pacing and Electrophysiology/British Pacing and Electrophysiology Group. Pacing Clin Electrophysiol 2002;25:260–4; with permission.

Table 2
North American Society for Pacing and Electrophysiology/British Pacing and Electrophysiology Group defibrillator code

Position I	Position II	Position III	Position IV
Shock Chambers(s)	ATP Chamber(s)	Tachycardia Detection	Antibradycardia Pacing Chamber(s)
O = None	O = None	E = Electrogram	O = None
A = Atrium	A = Atrium	H = Hemodynamic	A = Atrium
V = Ventricle	V = Ventricle		V = Ventricle
D = Dual (A + V)	D = Dual (A + V)		D = Dual (A + V)

From Bernstein AD, Camm AJ, Fisher JD, et al. North American Society of Pacing and Electrophysiology policy statement. The NASPE/BPEG defibrillator code. Pacing Clin Electrophysiol 1993;16:1776–80.

Malfunction stems from issues with the pulse generator or leads, or from external issues such as EMI–the most common cause during the perioperative period. Even when a properly functioning device is perceived to be malfunctioning (termed "pseudomalfunction"), harm to the patient and/or device can ensue; these events occur with some regularity in the hospital [29–31]. Although not well studied, for patients undergoing surgery, the presence of a CIED may be a risk factor for increased morbidity or mortality [11,12].

Thus, before elective surgery, a key step is ensuring that the patient's CIED is functioning properly, especially for surgery that is likely to result in hemodynamic embarrassment or whenever EMI (ie, which most commonly stems from the use of monopolar electrosurgery) is likely. Although there are no data conclusively showing the need for a comprehensive preoperative CIED evaluation, anecdotal evidence and case reports suggest that forgoing this step can result in adverse outcomes, including patient harm [19]. In any situation wherein a preoperative device evaluation cannot take place (see emergency surgery in later discussion), clinicians should be adequately prepared for perioperative device malfunction or failure that might occur [19].

Proper device function may often be established by querying the patient's medical record to determine when the CIED was last interrogated, and by accessing that interrogation report. The interrogation report should provide detailed information regarding the device type (ie, PM, ICD, CRT), the indication for its implantation, battery status, the current programming (including the magnet response), whether the patient is pacing dependent, and an overall assessment of whether the device was functioning properly at the time of the evaluation; often, a history of arrhythmias can be obtained. Typically, CIEDs should be evaluated every 3 to 12 months, with shorter intervals recommended for patients with more complicated devices (ie, CRT systems) or medical conditions, or devices under alert notification [14].

For instances in which previous records are not available or it is not otherwise possible to obtain information about the device, as previously noted, a CXR may be used to identify the device type, the device manufacturer (Fig. 8), and information about lead configuration. Additional steps that might

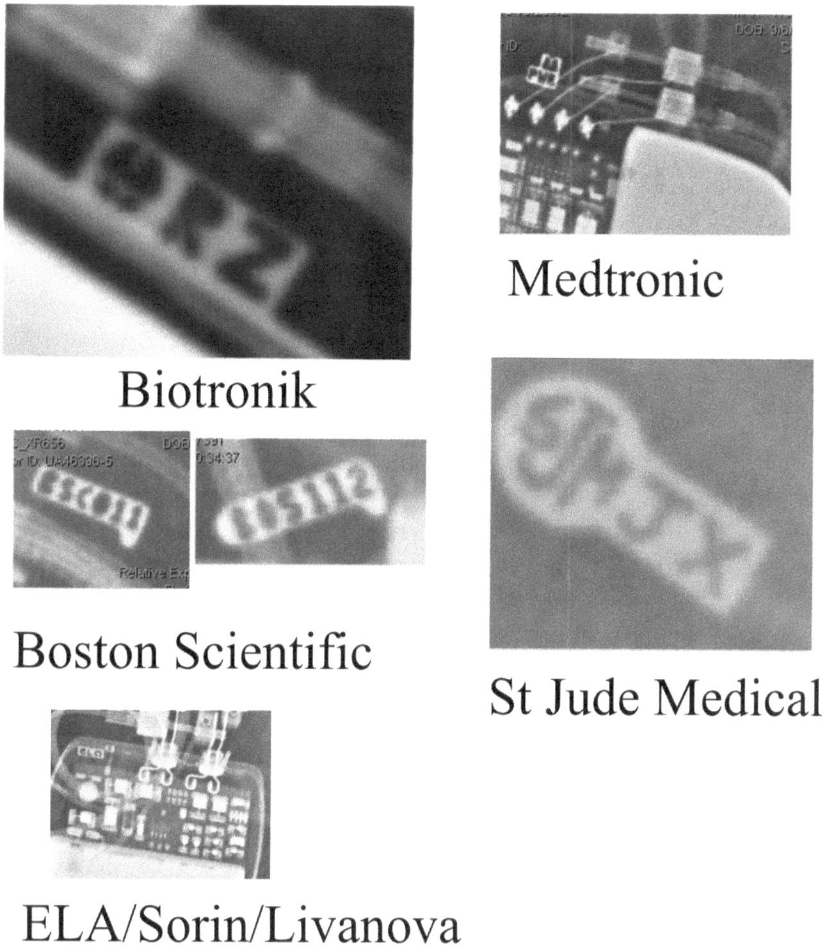

Fig. 8. Radiograph logos (*clockwise from upper left*): Biotronik (US Headquarters; Lake Oswego, OR), Medtronic, St Jude Medical, ELA 9 (which was purchased by Sorin [US Headquarters; Arvada, CO] and subsequently merged with Livanova [US Headquarters; Arvada, CO]), and Boston Scientific ("BSC" logo is most recent).

provide information about the device include reviewing the implant card that patients with CIED are instructed to carry with them at all times and calling the device manufacturer. Table 3 lists o device manufacturers and their phone numbers.

The patient

After confirming appropriate device function, the next step in preparing the patient with CIED for surgery is determining the patient's underlying rate

Table 3
Pulse generator company phone numbers

Biotronik	800-547-0394	Medtronic	800-505-4636
Boston Scientific	800-227-3422	St Jude Cardiac Rhythm Management	800-722-3774
ELA Medical Became (Sorin) Now LIVANOVA	877-663-7674		

and rhythm, and whether the patient is pacing dependent, because EMI-induced pacing inhibition (Fig. 9) may result in severe bradycardia or asystole in such patients. In general, pacing dependence implies the lack of spontaneous ventricular activity when the CIED is temporarily programmed to the VVI (single-chamber ventricular) or DDI (dual chamber pacing and sensing, but inhibited mode only) mode (or AAI for single-chamber atrial devices) at the lowest programmable rate (Fig. 10). Pacing dependency might alternatively be established by reviewing the patient's history or by examining the surface ECG. Patients with a history of AV node ablation or prior placement of a temporary pacing lead should be assumed to be pacing dependent. If a CIED was implanted for a symptomatic bradyarrhythmia or syncope, the patient might also be pacing dependent. On the ECG, pacing dependence

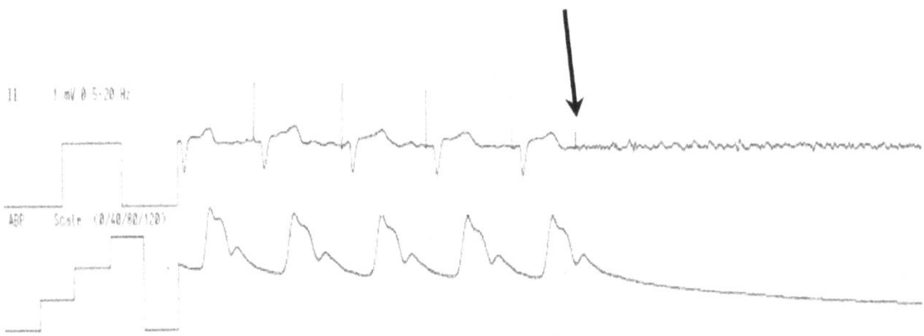

Fig. 9. Pacing inhibition from EMI leading to asystole in a pacing-dependent patient with third-degree heart block. A patient with persistent atrial fibrillation and a VVI PM set to 70 bpm was undergoing right total hip arthroplasty where monopolar electrosurgery was being conducted to a dispersive electrode on his upper back, allowing EMI to cause ventricular oversensing and pacing inhibition. (The preferred location for the dispersive electrode in this case would have been the thigh, ipsilateral to the surgical site.) The upper trace is ECG lead II, and the lower trace is the invasive arterial blood pressure. Pacing artifacts were being "painted" by the monitor electronics. Of note, the black downward arrow shows an inappropriately painted artifact caused by the monopolar electrosurgery interfering with the monitor pacing artifact detection, which explains the presumed "noncapture." Pacing resumed immediately upon cessation of monopolar ESU.

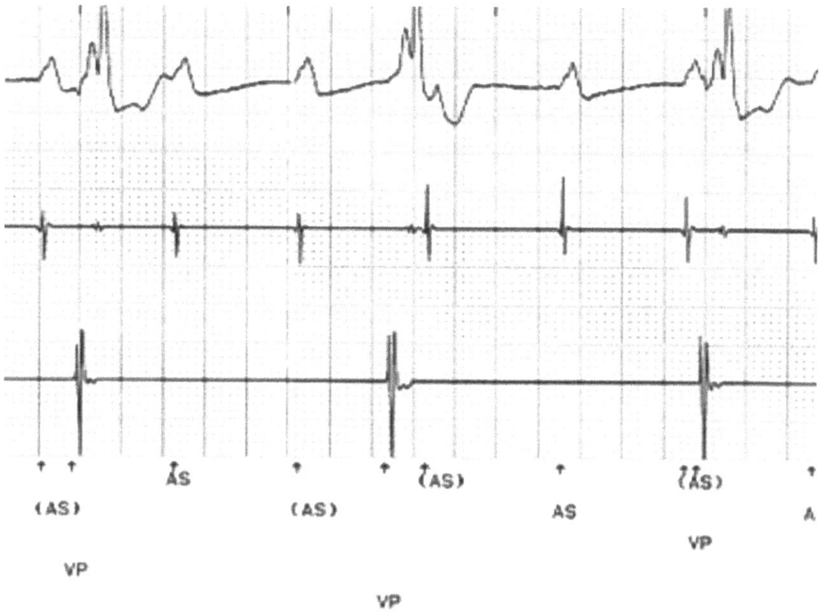

Fig. 10. Pacing dependence demonstrated during interrogation of underlying rhythm. This patient with a Boston Scientific PM was temporarily programmed to DDI at 40 bpm. He has an underlying sinus rhythm at 100 bpm and no conduction to the ventricles, rendering the designation of absolutely pacing dependent. The top trace is lead 2; the middle trace is the intracardiac signal from the atrial lead, and the bottom trace is the intracardiac signal from the right ventricular lead. The PM also provides its interpretation of the signals. "AS" means atrial sense (native atrial events are occurring at 600 milliseconds showing the sinus rhythm with rate 100 bpm). "VP" means ventricular pace. Note that no atrial event results in a conducted ventricular event (which would be labeled "VS.") This PM marks any atrial event preceded by an atrial event without an intervening ventricular event "(AS)."

should be assumed if every complex is paced, except for patients with a CRT device, because the goal of CRT programming is to force 100% biventricular pacing.

In general, the presence of a conventional CIED (ie, PM or ICD) does not necessitate special preoperative laboratory tests (that is, CXR, cardiac stress test, or echocardiogram). However, consideration should be given to obtaining a CXR in patients with suspected CIED malfunction, abandoned hardware, or leads on alert. Also, in the patient with a CRT device, documenting the position of the CS lead with a CXR before surgery might be useful, especially if central venous cannulation is planned, because spontaneous CS lead dislodgement can occur [32].

As for any surgical patient, proper management of the patient with CIED scheduled for an elective procedure always includes evaluation and optimization of coexisting disease. Although, as a general principle, the decision for preoperative testing should be based on non-CIED factors, such as the presence of medical comorbidities and stability of underlying disease, certain CIED-related conditions might prompt testing. For example, patients with an ICD or CRT device often have concomitant cardiomyopathy, heart failure, or other coexisting cardiovascular disease–conditions that might trigger a more extensive workup.

The procedure

Mitigating the effects of intraoperative EMI is the principal procedural concern. Thus, a key step to preoperative management is determining whether intraoperative EMI is anticipated so that appropriate precautions may be taken. In the operating room, ESU use is the most frequent cause of EMI, and monopolar electrosurgery is much more likely to cause EMI than bipolar electrosurgery [33]. In addition, the coagulation (high-voltage) mode causes more EMI than the nonblended cutting (low-voltage) mode [34]. The risk is greatest when the ESU will be used near the CIED pulse generator or leads and is typically considered significant when surgery is performed superior to the umbilicus [14,33]. Other important but less common sources of EMI [35–37] during the perioperative period include nerve stimulators for nerve blocks or peripheral nerve stimulation [38–40], transcutaneous electrical nerve stimulation [41–43], radiofrequency scanners used to find retained surgical instruments [44,45], lithotripsy, and other radiofrequency ablation machines or bone saws that cause vibration [46,47]. The ASA Practice Advisory states that all ICDs should have antitachycardia therapy disabled whenever monopolar ESU use is planned [15], whereas the HRS Expert Consensus Statement says ICD deactivation might not be needed when monopolar ESU will only be applied inferior to the patient's umbilicus [14]. Both the ASA and the HRS documents agree that consideration should be given to reprogramming any CIED to an asynchronous pacing mode for a pacing-dependent patient undergoing a procedure likely to cause EMI, and both statements caution that magnet application to an ICD cannot be used to accomplish this goal [14,15] (see later discussion on intraoperative management).

Additional considerations

In addition to suspending antitachycardia therapy and programming the CIED to an asynchronous pacing mode, before surgery additional changes to the device are sometimes warranted, including programming minute ventilation rate response (and possibly other pacing features that can mimic pacing system malfunction) to off when present, and changing the lower rate limit (ie, pacing rate) to optimize oxygen delivery (especially for major surgery).

INTRAOPERATIVE MANAGEMENT

No specific monitoring or anesthesia technique is required for the patient with CIED; however, the presence of a CIED does create specific intraoperative considerations.

Monitoring

Although standard ASA monitors (including continuous ECG, pulse oximetry, and capnography) are always required, every case in which the patient has a CIED also must include direct detection of mechanical systoles, because both EMI and the nerve stimulators used to monitor neuromuscular block can interfere with QRS complex display as well as detection and display of PM artifacts [34,37]. Most ECG monitors require reconfiguration of high-frequency filtering to demonstrate pacing pulses; however, ECG monitors can misinterpret pacing pulses as QRS complexes and display a nonzero heart rate for an asystolic patient [17]. Mechanical systoles are best evaluated by pulse oximetry plethysmography or invasive arterial pressure waveform display, and at least one these monitoring modalities is recommended for these cases by both that ASA and HRS advisories [14,15]. Inappropriate "painting" of pulse oximetry "systoles" can also occur; such false systoles reportedly led to a delay in the diagnosis of a cardiac arrest [48] (see Fig. 9).

Anesthetic agents

Drugs that suppress underlying rhythms, such as high-potency opiates [49] or dexmedetomidine [50], might render a pacing nondependent patient pacing dependent [51], thus reducing any margin of safety for pacing system failure. Anesthetic gases, such as isoflurane, sevoflurane, and desflurane, might prolong QT intervals, whereas halothane appears to reduce this interval [52–56].

Electromagnetic interference

As previously mentioned, during a surgical procedure, the function of a CIED may be impaired by EMI, and monopolar electrosurgery (ESU) use is the most prevalent source of intraoperative EMI. The risk of EMI from bipolar ESU is minimal. CIEDs with a unipolar electrode sensing configuration are more prone to EMI than those with a bipolar sensing configuration. Coagulation ESU will likely cause more problems than nonblended "cutting" ESU [33,34].

Several potential adverse consequences of EMI are possible; however, the 2 most common issues are (1) pacing inhibition and (2) delivery of inappropriate high-voltage therapy (ie, shocks or ATP). All CIEDs interpret electrical signals delivered through the electrodes as P or R waves. Pacing inhibition can occur when the CIED senses electrical activity (ie, electrosurgery "noise," myopotentials, T waves) that it should ignore but instead interprets as an intrinsic rhythm. Consequently, sometimes pacing inhibition in a pacing-dependent patient can result in profound bradycardia or asystole (see Fig. 9). If electrical activity is misinterpreted by an ICD as a tachyarrhythmia, inappropriate shocks or ATP might be triggered (Fig. 11), with the potential for serious consequences. The delivery of high-voltage therapy appears to release troponin [57], and even low-voltage ATP appears to injure the myocardium [58]. Both ATP and shock, whether appropriately delivered to treat a malignant ventricular arrhythmia or inappropriately delivered (ie, because of atrial fibrillation, another supraventricular rhythm, or EMI), have been associated with increased mortality [58]. In-hospital EMI appears to be responsible for more

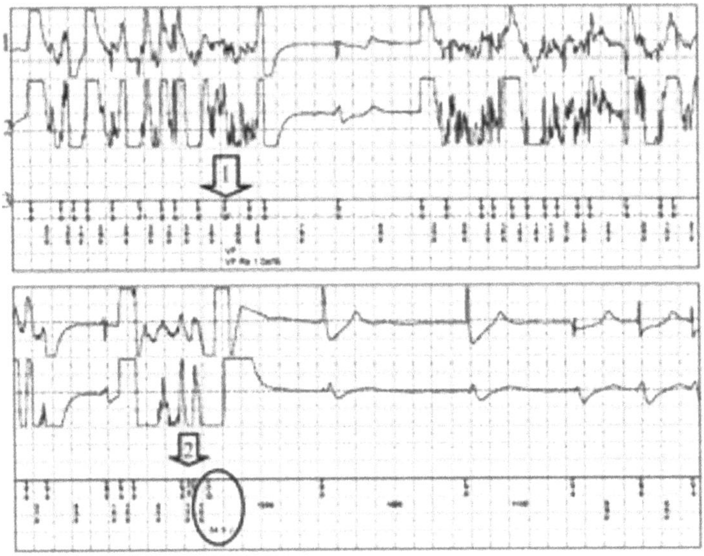

Fig. 11. Intraoperative EMI from monopolar electrosurgery leading to an inappropriate ICD shock. The electrogram demonstrates that a short burst of monopolar electrosurgery at an inopportune time caused the ICD to misdiagnose EMI as a malignant rhythm and deliver a 34.9-J shock. Trace "1" (*top panel*) reports the RV signal from the RV tip to ring electrodes. Trace "2" reports the RV signal collected using the RV ring electrode and the ICD "can." Trace "3" reports the ICD interpretation (marker channel) of the events (see legend below). At downward arrow "1," the ICD determined the aberrant signal persisted long enough to declare a ventricular fibrillation event "FD" and charge the capacitor in preparation for shock. ATP while charging was not delivered owing to several short RR intervals preceding charge initiation (this ICD will not deliver ATP while charging when any RR interval in the 8 proceeding RR intervals before the VF detection is <240 milliseconds). "CE" downward arrow "2" marks the end of capacitor charging and the start of VF reconfirm. Then, a very brief EMI event caused the 34.9-J charge delivery ("CD"). Because the EMI ("VF") stopped, the ICD classified this shock as successful termination of VF. The lack of EMI right after VF was declared too short to abort this event given the patient's native heart rate of about 80 bpm. CE, charge end; CD, charge delivered-cardioversion/defibrillation pulse; FD, VF detection; FS, VF sense; TS, VT sense; VP, ventricular pace; VS, ventricular sense.

than 4% of inappropriate shock therapy [59], which occurs in 20% to 40% of patients with ICDs [60,61].

Other adverse effects of EMI include (1) oversensing on the atrial lead, which, in a dual chamber pacing mode, can lead to right ventricular pacing at the upper tracking rate; (2) pacing at the upper sensor rate if the device has an active minute ventilation sensor, possibly leading to iatrogenic patient injury [29]; (3) "power on reset" wherein the device reverts to safety parameters, which include aggressive settings for ICD high-energy delivery and single-chamber pacing between 60 and 72.5 bpm regardless of the previous setting [14]; and (4) outright failure with no output. Because of the rare but catastrophic risk of outright failure, St Jude Medical has warned that pacing-dependent patients with legacy devices should undergo placement of temporary pacing backup in the setting of monopolar ESU use [62].

When intraoperative EMI is anticipated, specific actions are required to mitigate the associated risks. For an ICD, anti-tachyarrhythmia therapy should be disabled whenever EMI is likely or, even in the absence of anticipated EMI, if movement from a shock might create a hazard to the patient (ie, intraocular surgery) or procedural personnel (ie, hand surgery using a scalpel). During any period in which the ICD's anti-tachyarrhythmia therapy is disabled, ECG monitoring and the ability to deliver external cardioversion or defibrillation must be present. The ASA states that all ICDs should have anti-tachyarrhythmia therapy disabled whenever monopolar ESU use is planned, whereas the HRS states that ICD deactivation might not be needed for monopolar ESU application inferior to the umbilicus. Both the ASA and the HRS documents agree that consideration should be given to reprogramming a CIED to an asynchronous pacing mode for the pacing-dependent patient undergoing a procedure likely to cause EMI, and both statements caution that magnet application to an ICD does not accomplish this goal.

Caution must be observed with the use of invasive nerve stimulators when performing nerve blocks, because these devices can create EMI leading to ventricular oversensing (and therefore, pacing inhibition) as well [38,40].

Application of a surface nerve stimulator for neuromuscular monitoring within the CIED sensing axis can also inhibit pacing by producing pacing inhibition [63]. Transcutaneous nerve stimulators have also been implicated in the delivery of inappropriate high-energy therapy from an ICD [64]. Special testing is required in the setting of permanent nerve stimulator placement into any patient with a CIED, which is beyond the scope of this document [43].

The use of radiofrequency scanning (RFS) for retained instruments might also create EMI issues in patients with CIED [44,45]. CIED reprogramming before RFS might be indicated, and failure to alert anesthesiology personnel to initiation of RFS can result in asystole [44]. Whether operating room personnel with a CIED are at risk remains to be seen [65].

Finally, procedural personnel should be aware of mechanical issues that can cause a CIED to "detect" exercise, leading to an increase in pacing rates for rate responsive devices. Skin preparation in chest, head and neck, and upper extremity cases can produce vibratory effects that will induce increases in the "sensor indicated rate," a parameter internal to the CIED but which denotes the current lower pacing limit in an active rate response situation. External pressure on the CIED case [66,67] as well as bone saws applied to a site distal to the chest have caused pacing-driven tachycardias [47,68] to the upper sensor rate and confused perioperative personnel regarding the reason for the tachycardia.

Magnets

The decision whether to reprogram a CIED with a programming machine or to use a magnet instead depends on the type of CIED (PM or ICD), how it is programmed, the patient's underlying rhythm, the likelihood of EMI, the proximity of the CIED to the surgical field, and the planned patient positioning during surgery (eg, appropriate magnet application can be difficult or impossible in a patient who is in the prone or lateral position).

If magnet application is planned, the PM or ICD's magnet response should be known. For most transvenous PMs, magnet application will initiate asynchronous pacing at a fixed rate (85–100 bpm) as well as a fixed AV delay (as short as 100 milliseconds), which varies by manufacturer (and sometimes model) and which might not be appropriate for a given patient. For most transvenous ICDs, magnet application will suspend anti-tachyarrhythmia detection and/or therapy. However, some transvenous CIEDs can be programmed to respond differently to a magnet or have no response at all. Also, as previously stated, a magnet will never change the pacing mode of an ICD (ie, pacing inhibition may still occur). Moreover, if the sterile surgical field will include the CIED, then magnet application is usually not an option and the device will require reprogramming. Because CIED technology continues to evolve, expectations about magnet use will need to change. For example, magnet application to a Medtronic Micra leadless PM has no effect (by design) and is not programmable. Magnet application to a St Jude Nanostim leadless PM initiates VOO pacing at the 100/min for 8 cycles, 90/min assuming battery status normal, 65/min if battery status is "elective replacement indicated," assuming that the magnet sensor is programmed "ON."

Because of the aforementioned considerations, significant controversy exists regarding the appropriateness of using a magnet to achieve asynchronous pacing (PM) or temporarily suspend anti-tachyarrhythmia therapy (ICD). Although in many centers intraoperative magnet use is standard practice, and this approach is often advocated, magnet application may be unreliable, and several investigators have specifically warned against substituting the blind use of a magnet for individualized care. In a published series describing cases from 3 institutions, inadequate preoperative assessment of CIED function coupled with erroneous assumptions about the effects of magnet application contributed to or caused inappropriate ICD therapy, premature CIED battery depletion, and patient injury [19]. The investigators concluded that practitioners should exercise caution when applying magnets to CIEDs for surgery. Moreover, the practice of blindly placing a magnet over an ICD (ie, using a magnet and forgoing appropriate preoperative CIED evaluation) is discouraged by both the ASA and HRS.

Electrosurgical unit dispersive electrode placement

The dispersive electrode of the ESU should be placed such that the presumed current path from the ESU hand tool to the dispersive electrode (often incorrectly called "ground pad") does not cross the pulse generator or leads [33]. No data have been published regarding the safety of a whole-body dispersive electrode. The "harmonic scalpel," an ultrasonic cutting device, has been championed to prevent EMI while providing the surgeon with the ability to both cut and coagulate tissue. There are several case reports demonstrating successful surgery without EMI issues in these patients [69–71].

Additional considerations

Although many recommendations exist for external defibrillator pad placement to protect the ICD, one should remember that the patient, not the ICD, is being treated, and the anterior-posterior position remains favored. At some centers, the defibrillator pad is placed on the back, but not the front, of the ICD in the patient undergoing a procedure wherein the anterior pad would interfere with the procedure; thus, should an emergency arise, the anterior pad can be placed quickly and without significant repositioning of the patient.

POSTOPERATIVE MANAGEMENT

Many patients require postoperative CIED interrogation or reprogramming. In particular, any CIED that underwent preoperative or intraoperative reprogramming should be reinterrogated and have its parameters restored or optimized for perioperative recovery. Postoperative CIED interrogation should always be prompted by intraoperative hemodynamic instability or any concern for inappropriate CIED function. In many cases, rate enhancements may need to be reinitiated, and optimum heart rate and pacing parameters should be determined and ensured. The ICD patient must remain in a fully monitored setting (postanesthesia care unit or intensive care unit) until antitachycardia therapy is restored.

SUMMARY

The presence of an implantable PM or ICD (collectively, CIED) often complicates perioperative care and might even increase perioperative risk. These devices are being encountered in surgical patients with increasing frequency. Considerations in the proper care of the patient with CIED for surgery include (1) establishing communication with the patient's CIED physician, service, or other CIED expert to ensure appropriate CIED function; (2) acquiring knowledge about the CIED and how it is programmed to understand its intended function; (3) informing the patient's CIED physician, service, or other CIED expert of the upcoming surgical procedure and developing an appropriate perioperative CIED management plan; (4) enacting the perioperative management plan, which might include disabling an ICD's antitachycardia therapy, and asynchronous pacing for the pacing-dependent patient. All perioperative personnel must be made aware of the CIED, especially if electrical equipment (commonly monopolar electrosurgery) will be used that could interfere with CIED function. Whenever a preoperative device evaluation cannot take place or appropriate preoperative and/or intraoperative precautions cannot be enacted, clinicians should understand that device malfunction or failure might occur.

References

[1] Schulman PM, Rozner MA, Sera V, et al. Patients with pacemaker or implantable cardioverter-defibrillator. Med Clin North Am 2013;97(6):1051–75.
[2] Mond HG, Proclemer A. The 11th world survey of cardiac pacing and implantable cardioverter-defibrillators: calendar year 2009–a World Society of Arrhythmia's project. Pacing Clin Electrophysiol 2011;34(8):1013–27.
[3] Greenspon AJ, Patel JD, Lau E, et al. Trends in permanent pacemaker implantation in the United States from 1993 to 2009: increasing complexity of patients and procedures. J Am Coll Cardiol 2012;60(16):1540–5.
[4] Kurtz SM, Ochoa JA, Lau E, et al. Implantation trends and patient profiles for pacemakers and implantable cardioverter defibrillators in the United States: 1993-2006. Pacing Clin Electrophysiol 2010;33(6):705–11.
[5] Kremers MS, Hammill SC, Berul CI, et al. The National ICD Registry Report: version 2.1 including leads and pediatrics for years 2010 and 2011. Heart Rhythm 2013;10(4): e59–65.
[6] Schoenfeld MH. Contemporary pacemaker and defibrillator device therapy: challenges confronting the general cardiologist. Circulation 2007;115(5):638–53.
[7] Vetter TR, Ivankova NV, Goeddel LA, et al. An analysis of methodologies that can be used to validate if a perioperative surgical home improves the patient-centeredness, evidence-based practice, quality, safety, and value of patient care. Anesthesiology 2013;119(6): 1261–74.
[8] Rozner MA, Schulman PM. Creating an anesthesiologist-run pacemaker and defibrillator service: closing the perioperative care gap for these patients. Anesthesiology 2015;123(5):990–2.
[9] Russo AM. Are we improving care of Medicare patients undergoing primary prevention implantable cardioverter-defibrillator implantation? Circulation 2014;130:808–10.
[10] Pokorney SD, Miller AL, Chen AY, et al. Implantable cardioverter-defibrillator use among Medicare patients with low ejection fraction after acute myocardial infarction. JAMA 2015;313:2433–40.
[11] Badrinath SS, Bhaskaran S, Sundararaj I, et al. Mortality and morbidity associated with ophthalmic surgery. Ophthalmic Surg Lasers 1995;26(6):535–41.
[12] Pili-Floury S, Farah E, Samain E, et al. Perioperative outcome of pacemaker patients undergoing non-cardiac surgery. Eur J Anaesthesiol 2008;25(6):514–6.
[13] Cima RR, Brown MJ, Hebl JR, et al. Use of lean and six sigma methodology to improve operating room efficiency in a high-volume tertiary-care academic medical center. J Am Coll Surg 2011;213(1):83–92 [discussion: 3–4].
[14] Crossley GH, Poole JE, Rozner MA, et al. The Heart Rhythm Society (HRS)/American Society of Anesthesiologists (ASA) Expert Consensus Statement on the perioperative management of patients with implantable defibrillators, pacemakers and arrhythmia monitors: facilities and patient management this document was developed as a joint project with the American Society of Anesthesiologists (ASA), and in collaboration with the American Heart Association (AHA), and the Society of Thoracic Surgeons (STS). Heart Rhythm 2011;8(7):1114–54.
[15] American Society of Anesthesiologists. Practice advisory for the perioperative management of patients with cardiac implantable electronic devices: pacemakers and implantable cardioverter-defibrillators: an updated report by the American Society of Anesthesiologists task force on perioperative management of patients with cardiac implantable electronic devices. Anesthesiology 2011;114(2):247–61.
[16] Healey JS, Merchant R, Simpson C, et al. Society position statement: Canadian Cardiovascular Society/Canadian Anesthesiologists' Society/Canadian Heart Rhythm Society joint position statement on the perioperative management of patients with implanted pacemakers, defibrillators, and neurostimulating devices. Can J Anaesth 2012;59:394–407.

[17] Guidelines for the perioperative management of patients with implantable pacemakers or implantable cardioverter defibrillators, where the use of surgical diathermy/electrocautery is anticipated. Medicines and Health Care Products Regulatory Agency; 2006. Available at: https://www.erbe-med.com/images/uk/Diathermy__Pacemakers-ICDs1.pdf. Accessed May 5, 2015.
[18] Naccarelli GV, Conti JB, DiMarco JP, et al. Task force 6: training in specialized electrophysiology, cardiac pacing, and arrhythmia management endorsed by the Heart Rhythm Society. J Am Coll Cardiol 2008;51(3):374–80.
[19] Schulman PM, Rozner MA. Case report: use caution when applying magnets to pacemakers or defibrillators for surgery. Anesth Analg 2013;117(2):422–7.
[20] Epstein AE, DiMarco JP, Ellenbogen KA, et al. ACC/AHA/HRS 2008 guidelines for device-based therapy of cardiac rhythm abnormalities: a report of the American College of Cardiology/American Heart Association Task Force on Practice Guidelines (writing committee to revise the ACC/AHA/NASPE 2002 guideline update for implantation of cardiac pacemakers and Antiarrhythmia Devices): developed in collaboration with the American Association for Thoracic Surgery and Society of Thoracic Surgeons. Circulation 2008;117: e350–408.
[21] Rowley CP, Gold MR. Subcutaneous implantable cardioverter defibrillator. Circ Arrhythm Electrophysiol 2012;5:587–93 [review].
[22] Bernstein AD, Daubert JC, Fletcher RD, et al. The revised NASPE/BPEG generic code for antibradycardia, adaptive-rate, and multisite pacing. North American Society of Pacing and Electrophysiology/British Pacing and Electrophysiology Group. Pacing Clin Electrophysiol 2002;25(2):260–4.
[23] Bernstein AD, Camm AJ, Fisher JD, et al. North American Society of Pacing and Electrophysiology policy statement. The NASPE/BPEG defibrillator code. Pacing Clin Electrophysiol 1993;16:1776–80.
[24] Rozner MA, Schulman PM. How should we prepare the patient with a pacemaker/implantable cardioverter-defibrillator?. In: Fleisher LA, editor. Evidence-based practice of anesthesiology. 3rd edition. Philadelphia: Saunders; 2013. p. 88–97.
[25] Tseng ZH, Hayward RM, Clark NM, et al. Sudden death in patients with cardiac implantable electronic devices. JAMA Intern Med 2015;175(8):1342–50.
[26] Gornick CC, Hauser RG, Almquist AK, et al. Unpredictable implantable cardioverter-defibrillator pulse generator failure due to electrical overstress causing sudden death in a young high-risk patient with hypertrophic cardiomyopathy. Heart Rhythm 2005;2:2681–3.
[27] Maisel WH, Moynahan M, Zuckerman BD, et al. Pacemaker and ICD generator malfunctions: analysis of Food and Drug Administration annual reports. JAMA 2006;295(16): 1901–6.
[28] Laskey W, Awad K, Lum J, et al. An analysis of implantable cardiac device reliability. The case for improved postmarketing risk assessment and surveillance. Am J Ther 2012;19(4):248–54.
[29] Lau W, Corcoran SJ, Mond HG. Pacemaker tachycardia in a minute ventilation rate-adaptive pacemaker induced by electrocardiographic monitoring. Pacing Clin Electrophysiol 2006;29:438–40.
[30] Rozner MA, Nishman RJ. Pacemaker-driven tachycardia revisited. Anesth Analg 1999;88:965.
[31] Rozner MA, Nishman RJ. Electrocautery-induced pacemaker tachycardia: why does this error continue? Anesthesiology 2002;96:773–4.
[32] Biffi M, Bertini M, Ziacchi M, et al. Left ventricular lead stabilization to retain cardiac resynchronization therapy at long term: when is it advisable? Europace 2014;16:533–40.
[33] Robinson TN, Varosy PD, Guillaume G, et al. Effect of radiofrequency energy emitted from monopolar "Bovie" instruments on cardiac implantable electronic devices. J Am Coll Surg 2014;219(3):399–406.

[34] Rozner MA. Review of electrical interference in implanted cardiac devices. Pacing Clin Electrophysiol 2003;26(4 Pt 1):923–5.
[35] Rozner MA. Pacemaker and electrocardiographic monitor psuedomalfunction during extracardiac radiofrequency ablation. Anesthesiology 2005;102:239.
[36] Rozner MA. Peripheral nerve stimulators can inhibit monitor display of pacemaker pulses. J Clin Anesth 2004;16:117–20.
[37] Rozner MA. Peripheral nerve stimulators can inhibit monitor display of pacemaker pulses. J Clin Anesth 2004;16(2):117–20.
[38] Engelhardt L, Große J, Birnbaum J, et al. Inhibition of a pacemaker during nerve stimulation for regional anaesthesia. Anaesthesia 2007;62(10):1071–4.
[39] Ducey JP, Fincher CW, Baysinger CL. Therapeutic suppression of a permanent ventricular pacemaker using a peripheral nerve stimulator. Anesthesiology 1991;75:533.
[40] McKay RE, Rozner MA. Preventing pacemaker problems with nerve stimulators. Anaesthesia 2008;63:554.
[41] Occhetta E, Bortnik M, Magnani A, et al. Inappropriate implantable cardioverter-defibrillator discharges unrelated to supraventricular tachyarrhythmias. Europace 2006;8:863.
[42] Carlson T, Andréll P, Ekre O, et al. Interference of transcutaneous electrical nerve stimulation with permanent ventricular stimulation: a new clinical problem? Europace 2009;11:364.
[43] Molon G, Perrone C, Maines M, et al. ICD and neuromodulation devices: is peaceful coexistence possible? Pacing Clin Electrophysiol 2011;34(6):690–3.
[44] Plakke MJ, Maisonave Y, Daley SM. Radiofrequency scanning for retained surgical items can cause electromagnetic interference and pacing inhibition if an asynchronous pacing mode is not applied. A A Case Rep 2016;6(6):143–5.
[45] Seidman SJ, Brockman R, Lewis BM, et al. In vitro tests reveal sample radiofrequency identification readers inducing clinically significant electromagnetic interference to implantable pacemakers and implantable cardioverter-defibrillators. Heart Rhythm 2010;7(1):99–107.
[46] Varma N, Cunningham D, Falk R. Central venous access resulting in selective failure of ICD defibrillation capacity. Pacing Clin Electrophysiol 2001;24:394.
[47] Schwartzenburg CF, Wass CT, Strickland RA, et al. Rate-adaptive cardiac pacing: implications of environmental noise during craniotomy. Anesthesiology 1997;87:1252.
[48] Kuroda M, Kawamoto M, Yuge O. Undisrupted pulse wave on pulse oximeter display monitor at cardiac arrest in a surgical patient. J Anesth 2005;19:164–6.
[49] Arnold RW, Jensen PA, Kovtoun TA, et al. The profound augmentation of the oculocardiac reflex by fast acting opioids. Binocul Vis Strabismus Q 2004;19:215–22.
[50] Gerlach AT, Murphy CV, Dasta JF. An updated focused review of dexmedetomidine in adults. Ann Pharmacother 2009;43:2064.
[51] Healey JS, Merchant R, Simpson C, et al. Canadian Cardiovascular Society/Canadian Anesthesiologists' Society/Canadian Heart Rhythm Society joint position statement on the perioperative management of patients with implanted pacemakers, defibrillators, and neurostimulating devices. Can J Cardiol 2012;28:141.
[52] Michaloudis D, Fraidakis O, Petrou A, et al. Anaesthesia and the QT interval. Effects of isoflurane and halothane in unpremedicated children. Anaesthesia 1998;53:435.
[53] Michaloudis D, Fraidakis O, Lefaki T, et al. Anaesthesia and the QT interval in humans: effects of halothane and isoflurane in premedicated children. Eur J Anaesthesiol 1998;15:623.
[54] Gallagher JD, Weindling SN, Anderson G, et al. Effects of sevoflurane on QT interval in a patient with congenital long QT syndrome. Anesthesiology 1998;89:1569.
[55] Paventi S, Santevecchi A, Ranieri R. Effects of sevoflurane versus propofol on QT interval. Minerva Anestesiol 2001;67:637.
[56] Yildirim H, Adanir T, Atay A, et al. The effects of sevoflurane, isoflurane and desflurane on QT interval of the ECG. Eur J Anaesthesiol 2004;21:566.
[57] Hasdemir C, Shah N, Rao AP, et al. Analysis of troponin I levels after spontaneous implantable cardioverter defibrillator shocks. J Cardiovasc Electrophysiol 2002;13:144–50.

[58] Stempniewicz P, Cheng A, Connolly A, et al. Appropriate and inappropriate electrical therapies delivered by an implantable cardioverter-defibrillator: effect on intracardiac electrogram. J Cardiovasc Electrophysiol 2011;22:554–60.
[59] Powell BD, Asirvatham SJ, Perschbacher DL, et al. Noise, artifact, and oversensing related inappropriate ICD shock evaluation: ALTITUDE noise study. Pacing Clin Electrophysiol 2012;35(7):863–9.
[60] Moss AJ, Schuger C, Beck CA, et al. Reduction in inappropriate therapy and mortality through ICD Programming. N Engl J Med 2012;367:2275–83.
[61] Atwater BD, Daubert JP. Implantable cardioverter defibrillators: risks accompany the life-saving benefits. Heart 2012;98:764–72.
[62] Considerations when using electrocautery in patients implanted with older generation St. Jude Medical pacemakers. St Jude Medical; 2014. Available at: https://www.sjm.com/~/media/galaxy/hcp/resources-reimbursement/technical-resources/product-adviseries-archive/stjude-pacemaker-notice-012914.pdf?la=en. Accessed May 6, 2016.
[63] Moskowitz DM, Kahn RA, Camunas J, et al. External chest wall stimulation to suppress a permanent transvenous pacemaker in a patient during endovascular stent graft placement. Anesthesiology 1998;89:531–3.
[64] Curwin JH, Coyne RF, Winters SL. Inappropriate defibrillator (ICD) shocks caused by transcutaneous electronic nerve stimulation (TENS) units. Pacing Clin Electrophysiol 1999;22:692–3.
[65] Rozner MA, Schultheis L, Schulman PM. The unstated Murphy's law of the operating room: if something goes wrong, blame anesthesia. A A Case Rep 2016;6:139–41.
[66] Altose M, Leon-Ruiz E. Etomidate-induced pacemaker-mediated ventricular tachycardia. Anesthesiology 2007;106:1059–60.
[67] Rozner MA. Etomidate unlikely to have induced pacemaker-mediated tachycardia. Anesthesiology 2007;107:1036–7.
[68] Levine PA. Response to "rate-adaptive cardiac pacing: implications of environmental noise during craniotomy". Anesthesiology 1997;87:1261.
[69] Nandalan SP, Vanner RG. Use of the harmonic scalpel in a patient with a permanent pacemaker. Anaesthesia 2004;59:621.
[70] Epstein MR, Mayer JE Jr, Duncan BW. Use of an ultrasonic scalpel as an alternative to electrocautery in patients with pacemakers. Ann Thorac Surg 1998;65:1802–4.
[71] Ozeren M, Dogan OV, Duzgun C, et al. Use of an ultrasonic scalpel in the open-heart reoperation of a patient with pacemaker. Eur J Cardiothorac Surg 2002;21:761–2.

Advances in Anesthesia 34 (2016) 143–160

ADVANCES IN ANESTHESIA

Evidence Basis and Practical Management of Postoperative Thoracic Epidural Analgesia

Michelle C. Parra, MD[a], Patricia J. Barr, RN[b], Mark P. Yeager, MD[b,*]

[a]Department of Anesthesia, University of Iowa Hospitals and Clinics, 200 Hawkins Drive, Iowa City, IA 52242, USA; [b]Department of Anesthesiology, Dartmouth-Hitchcock Medical Center, 1 Medical Center Drive, Lebanon, NH 03756, USA

Keywords

• Epidural analgesia • Pain, postoperative • Recovery, surgical
• Outcomes, surgical • Epidural catheter management

Key points

- Thoracic epidural analgesia (TEA) after major thoracic or abdominal surgery provides documented benefits that improve physiologic recovery and increase patient satisfaction.
- The decision to use TEA should be made in the context of rapidly changing practice protocols and alternative approaches that are designed to enhance the patient recovery process.
- The effectiveness of TEA is improved by dedicated protocols that include interventions to minimize catheter malfunction and side effects and maximize analgesic effectiveness.
- Thoracic epidural catheter management is a dynamic process that requires a balance of team-based protocols and ongoing patient-specific decision making.

EVOLUTION OF THORACIC EPIDURAL ANALGESIA

The current role of anesthetic management in surgical recovery was foreshadowed at the start of the twentieth century when George Crile, surgeon and a Cleveland Clinic founder, advocated his technique of "anoci-association" to

All authors declare no conflicts of interest or funding support for this article.

*Corresponding author. *E-mail address:* mark.p.yeager@hitchcock.org

http://dx.doi.org/10.1016/j.aan.2016.07.009
0737-6146/16/

improve surgical outcomes [1,2]. The parallels between Crile's approach to surgical recovery and current practice are remarkable:

Components of Crile's Anoci-association	Crile's approach Circa 1915	Current Approach Circa 2015
Minimize surgical trauma	Gentle manipulation, sharp dissection	Laparoscopic, robot-assisted surgery
Minimize patient stress response	Liberal injections of local anesthetic	Use of epidural and regional blocks
Minimize postoperative pain	Neurolytic blocks after surgery	Continuous catheter and multimodal analgesia techniques
Minimize effect of general anesthesia	Use nitrous oxide, avoid ether	Electroencephalogram-guided anesthesia, total intravenous anesthesia

During the 1930s and 1940s, Walter Cannon [3] and Hans Selye [4] provided the physiologic underpinnings for Crile's results with the introduction of their concepts of "homeostasis" and "stress," respectively. The next advance took place when what might be called the modern era of perioperative anesthetic management became a reality in the 1970s. By then administration of local anesthetics into the epidural space to provide surgical or obstetric anesthesia had been known for decades. In the 1970s, adoption of thoracic epidural anesthesia and TEA into clinical practice became a reality with (1) improvements in epidural catheter design, (2) case series reports of postoperative epidural analgesia [5,6], and (3) the publication of Bromage's classic textbook on epidural analgesia [7].

Shortly thereafter the introduction of neuraxial analgesia [8] and, more recently, the development of hospital-based acute pain services (APSs) [9] have furthered the popularity of TEA. With the constant and rapid introduction of new techniques and surgical approaches, TEA remains an evolving practice that requires continuous evaluation, re-evaluation, and adaptation.

CURRENT PRACTICE

Many profoundly important changes in surgical care have appeared in rapid succession coincident with changes in management of postoperative pain. Some of the more obvious developments that should be incorporated into a contemporary decision-making paradigm include

- Widespread use of laparoscopic and thoracoscopic techniques for major surgery
- Development of enhanced recovery after surgery (ERAS) protocols for specific procedures
- Acceptances of alternative techniques for postoperative analgesia, such as transversus abdominis plane (TAP) blocks and thoracic paraveterbral blocks
- Widespread use of ultrasound guidance to improve the efficacy of peripheral nerve blocks

- Peripheral nerve continuous catheter techniques for postoperative analgesia
- Introduction of long-acting local anesthetic formulations

Additionally, surgical outcomes have improved significantly in recent years [10], making it difficult to definitively assess the benefits of a single perioperative intervention. Despite these changes, TEA remains an important component of high-quality care during surgical recovery from many major procedures. The durability of TEA's popularity is a consequence of demonstrable clinical effectiveness for a variety of important outcomes, such as decreased postoperative mortality, cardiopulmonary morbidity, enhanced recovery of bowel function, opioid-sparing effects, earlier mobilization, and diminished hypercoagulability [11]. The ongoing popularity of TEA may also be a consequence of this consideration: although there are alternative approaches to regulating the individual components of a patient's surgical recovery, TEA is the only single intervention that improves the recovery profile for all these physiologic outcomes.

Finally, most clinicians work in an environment where real outcomes, such as major morbidity, mortality, length of hospital stay, and so forth, have taken on increased importance compared with so-called intermediate outcomes, such as pain control and pulmonary function. In this setting, TEA has become less of a stand-alone intervention and more of a companion to a variety of other therapies that are currently used to enhance the recovery process. This more inclusive use of TEA dictates ongoing reappraisals of TEA to streamline implementation, maximize effectiveness, and minimize side effects.

DOCUMENTED BENEFITS OF THORACIC EPIDURAL ANALGESIA FOR SURGICAL RECOVERY

Hundreds of clinical studies completed in recent years have examined specific benefits of TEA in defined surgical populations. Documented benefits have been shown for [11]

- Decreased mortality
- Improving pulmonary function and decreasing complications
- Decreasing cardiovascular morbidity
- Earlier recovery of bowel function
- Earlier patient mobilization
- Opioid sparing
- Neuroendocrine/immune responses to surgery
- Thromboembolic events
- Patient satisfaction

Pulmonary function and complications

Improvements in pulmonary function and prevention of pulmonary morbidity were the initial impetus for introducing TEA into clinical practice and several reviews on this subject have been published [12–15]. Overall, any type of neuraxial analgesia (epidural or intrathecal) using local anesthetic or a combination of local anesthetic and opioid is superior compared with systemic analgesia [12,16]. Clinicians should also note, however, that (1) the overall incidence of pulmonary complications seems to be declining, thus lowering the relative effectiveness of TEA [13], and (2) it is usually not possible to determine if a pulmonary benefit from TEA is due to superior analgesia via TEA or to an opioid-sparing effect (avoidance of sedation/hypoventilation). The latter observation has relevance for patients managed with multimodal analgesia regimens where opioid-sparing via mechanisms other than TEA is a primary objective. Additionally, a precise physiologic relationship between quality of analgesia and pulmonary function is difficult to demonstrate. In general, however, most clinicians have found (and the data demonstrate) that the more traumatic and invasive the surgery and the closer surgery is to the diaphragm, the greater the benefit of using TEA to minimize pulmonary complications [17–20].

Cardiovascular morbidity

The use of TEA to prevent cardiovascular morbidity and/or cardiac-related mortality remains somewhat controversial. Local anesthetic blockade of cardiac sympathetic innervation via upper thoracic sympathetic nerves can significantly improve myocardial oxygen supply/demand relationships in patients with coronary artery disease via several mechanisms [21]. As well, use of postoperative TEA diminishes the sympathetic activation associated with major surgery [22]. Direct application of these physiologic effects into clinical practice requires clinical judgment and context due to the wide variety of effective preoperative cardiac-specific interventions (eg, antiangina medications and coronary angioplasty) available to surgical patients. If TEA is used to minimize cardiac risk (ischemia, infarction, or arrhythmia), the evidence suggests that a thoracic (not lumbar) epidural catheter is effective [23] and the benefits are most apparent in patients at highest risk for such events (high risk of coronary artery disease and high-risk surgery) [17,24].

Recovery of bowel function

TEA, compared with systemic analgesia, leads to earlier recovery of bowel function after abdominal surgery [25–27]. Use of local anesthetic in the epidural solution is important and yields a better result than use of epidural opioid alone [28]. The mechanism for earlier recovery of bowel function (an effect that varies widely but is considerable in some studies [26]) is also not clear. It could be due to better pain control (reported by some studies), avoidance of opioid induced ileus, and/or abdominal sympatholysis with predominance of vagal innervation. Whatever the mechanism, it seems that this benefit requires an ongoing infusion of local anesthetic medication into the epidural catheter [29].

Patient mobilization

Patient mobilization as an indirect indicator for rate of postsurgical recovery, discharge, and, ultimately, resource utilization is the subject of increasing attention from clinicians, hospital administrators, and third-party payers. Two components of the process of postsurgical mobilization are demonstrably improved by TEA. First, pain with movement (dynamic pain) is improved with TEA compared with systemic analgesia [14,17,30]. The latter can provide comparable analgesic effects compared with TEA for pain at rest, but with movement TEA is superior. Second, TEA can diminish the negative nitrogen balance and protein breakdown that commonly accompany major thoracic or abdominal surgical trauma [31]. Optimizing pain control after major surgery also results in diminished patient reports of fatigue [32]. Thus, particularly when used in a multimodal approach to recovery, TEA decreases length of stay and increases patient satisfaction [20,33,34]. The specific contribution of TEA in these programs has not been isolated however, and may never be clarified due to the large number of variables and the dynamic, evolving nature of the clinical care environment [35].

Opioid sparing

Minimization of opioid use[a] is an essential part of enhanced recovery programs primarily for avoidance of common side effects: sedation, respiratory depression, constipation, nausea, delirium, immune suppression, and urinary retention. By minimizing opioid use, the incidence of these side effects is decreased [9]. TEA decreases overall opioid consumption, improves postsurgical pain scores [34], and is widely recommended for thoracic and major abdominal surgery [20,33,36]. When TEA is combined with multimodal analgesia, opioid use can often be avoided altogether. Although evidence to link postoperative pain control with surgical outcomes (other than patient satisfaction) is often difficult to demonstrate, evidence shows that better pain control certainly leads to better pulmonary outcomes [9]. Definitive conclusions about specific combinations of analgesic interventions is, however, difficult [37–39]. Opioid-sparing effects (with or without TEA) have been reported for

- Acetaminophen [38,39]
- Nonsteroidal anti-inflammatory drugs [40]
- Gabapentin/pregabalin [41]
- Ketamine [42]
- Glucocorticoids [37]
- Intravenous lidocaine [43]
- Tramadol [41]

Neuroendocrine/metabolic/immune response to surgery

The 1980s brought the introduction and widespread availability of serum ELISA assays that measure circulating mediators of the human stress response

[a]Is it safe to use systemic opioids (patient controlled analgesia [PCA]) with an epidural infusion? Provided a patient's condition does not suggest increased risk of respiratory depression (eg, obesity, obstructive sleep apnea, use of other sedative medications, advanced age, debility, etc.), the authors use epidural infusions (typically hydromorphone,10 μg/mL, or fentanyl, 2 μg/mL) with PCA but only under certain conditions: (1) assess level of sedation before and during administration of systemic opioids (see "Analgesic solutions") and (2) no basal/continuous PCA infusion unless approved by APS.

to surgical trauma. Studies were soon published that demonstrated a diminution in this response with regional anesthetic and analgesic techniques, especially TEA [44]. Although it is difficult to directly link control of the stress response to primary surgical outcomes, there are documented organ-specific benefits, such as avoiding tachycardia due to elevated catecholamines or catabolism associated with hypercortisolemia. Immune suppression after major surgery is another consequence of the stress response that may be minimized with TEA, either directly or via associated opioid-sparing effects, because opioids have been shown to suppress some measures of human immunity [45].

Thromboembolic events

The widely published guidelines regarding when it is safe to insert or remove an epidural catheter in a patient on anticoagulant or antiplatelet medications [46] are designed to minimize the risk of spinal hematoma formation and to address concerns of surgeons regarding untimely administration of deep vein thrombosis prophylaxis. These concerns somewhat overshadow a documented benefit that TEA can have on the risk of a thromboembolic event. Low thoracic or lumbar epidural anesthesia increases lower extremity blood flow, either as a consequence of vasodilation and/or avoidance of positive pressure ventilation [47]. In addition, epidural anesthesia was shown to decrease the incidence of thromboembolic events in high-risk surgery, such as hip surgery [48], and to decrease the incidence of early lower extremity vascular graft failure [49,50], either by the mechanisms discussed previously or by minimizing the hypercoagulability that often follows major surgery or by a systemic anti-inflammatory effect of epidurally administered local anesthetics [51,52].

Patient satisfaction

It is difficult to demonstrate that pain relief per se improves clinical outcomes, but when optimal analgesia is provided for postoperative patients, satisfaction improves [9]. Along with this observation, there are also data to suggest that improved acute pain management may decrease the incidence of persistent postoperative pain after surgery [32,42,53]. As an outcome, patient satisfaction is receiving increased attention and should, therefore, be part of the clinical decision-making process.

Potential side effects of thoracic epidural analgesia

Urinary retention and urinary tract infection

Urinary tract infections are a common hospital-acquired infection directly linked to the presence of an indwelling urinary catheter. Some practitioners continue to believe that an indwelling urinary catheter is necessary as long as TEA is ongoing to avoid urinary retention. Not only does this approach ignore the fact that systemic opioids can also cause urinary retention but also, more importantly, studies show that the incidence of urinary retention (defined as the need for recatheterization) is low (5%–8%) when TEA (distinct from lumbar epidural analgesia [LEA]) is used with dilute solutions of local anesthetics in patients who are otherwise at low risk for urinary retention

[34,54,55]. Early removal urinary catheter decreases the incidence of urinary tract infections [54].

Hypotension

Perhaps the most common and immediately worrisome side effect of TEA is hypotension, which may be a consequence of either direct vasodilation or, somewhat paradoxically, decreased pain. Although complete elimination of this side effect is probably not possible (especially if more effective pain control is part of the cause), it can be minimized by careful attention to fluid management during and after surgery. The best results are observed when protocols are in place to use either monitor-guided and goal-directed intravascular volume management [34] or specific protocols in which fluid administration is based on extent of surgical trauma [20,56]. When such protocols are combined with TEA infusion protocols that emphasize dilute solutions of local anesthetic (eg, 0.1%–0.0625% bupivacaine) the incidence of clinically significant hypotension is minimized. There are published data to suggest that a poorly functioning epidural catheter (inadequate analgesia) is not only more common but potentially just as dangerous as a well-functioning epidural catheter (that may induce hypotension) [57].

Muscle weakness

Early reports of epidural analgesia, especially LEA, reported lower extremity weakness as a side effect, but this was usually in conjunction with comparatively high concentrations of local anesthetic (0.25% bupivacaine, for example). With more widespread use of dilute solutions of local anesthetic and avoidance of LEA, lower extremity motor weakness is a rare side effect and should not impede mobilization. Analgesic effectiveness of dilute local anesthetic solutions can be improved with the addition of opioids to the epidural infusion (eg, hydromorphone, 10 μg/mL, or fentanyl, 2 μg/mL) and/or the addition of patient-controlled epidural analgesia (PCEA) to a continuous epidural infusion.

Severe complications

Severe complications associated with TEA are rare [58]. The rare but severe complications of clinically significant respiratory depression, infection, and epidural/spinal hematoma remain a concern in all patients. Guidelines to minimize the incidence of both have been published [46,59].

THORACIC EPIDURAL ANALGESIA INDICATIONS AND ALTERNATIVES

Which patients clearly benefit from TEA and which benefit from an alternative approach (Table 1)? The surgical procedure and the presence of comorbidities are the primary considerations that help answer this question. Surgery of the thorax (open or thoracoscopic) and upper abdominal and major lower abdominal (urologic and gynecologic) procedures usually benefit from TEA. Patients with pulmonary comorbidities have the most proved benefit due to better analgesia during dynamic movements–respiratory effort and coughing, leading to

Table 1
Thoracic epidural analgesia benefits and drawbacks

Type of block	Procedure	Benefits	Drawbacks
Epidural	Open thoracic or major abdominal	Multiply with ↑ comorbidities	Placement time Failure rate
Epidural	Minimally invasive: thoracic or abdominal	None proved	Side effects
TAP block	(Lower) abdominal	Reliability	Limited coverage and duration
Paravertebral	Thoracic, breast	Unilateral, minimize TEA side effects	Placement time Requires specific training
Spinal	Minimally invasive abdominal Joint arthroplasty	High success rate	Limited duration

fewer pulmonary complications. Patients with centrally mediated or obstructive sleep apnea who are sensitive to sedating effects of opioids and general anesthetics also benefit because TEA reduces opioid requirements. Avoiding sedating medications is also important for the elderly at risk for postoperative cognitive dysfunction. Studies have yet to clearly associate anesthetic and analgesic technique with postoperative cognitive dysfunction [60], but there is consensus that reduction in perioperative medication consumption (opioids) should improve overall postoperative cognitive health. Patients with a history of medication allergies, especially adverse reactions to opioids, also benefit. TEA works well when incorporated into enhanced recovery protocols, such as for colorectal surgery, where the earlier return of postoperative bowel function is important [14,61].

The TAP block is an alternative to TEA for some patients. The TAP block was described in 2001 [62] and popularized with the introduction of ultrasound guidance for correct placement of local anesthetic solution [63]. TAP blocks are a field block in the fascial plane between the internal oblique and transversus abdominis muscle layers on the lateral abdominal wall. A TAP block creates a unilateral, approximately T10-L1, dermatomal distribution of analgesia after injection of 20-mL dilute local anesthetic. Benefits include reduction in postoperative opioid consumption, lower pain scores, and fewer opioid side effects. TAP blocks are most effective for Pfannenstiel-type incisions, infraumbilical vertical abdominal incisions, and small unilateral incisions associated with ileostomy creation/takedown or inguinal hernia repair. A subcostal approach with injection of local anesthetic at a more cephalad dermatome level can provide analgesia for incisions above the umbilicus [64]. A TAP block may also be applicable in the ambulatory patient population providing effective analgesia from a single injection after short outpatient procedures associated with mild to moderate postoperative pain.

Another TEA alternative is a thoracic paravertebral block, which was (re) introduced into common practice after the description of a catheter-based technique [65]. Paravertebral blocks create somatic sensory and sympathetic blockade that involves approximately 5 and 8 dermatomal levels, respectively, after a 15-mL injection of local anesthetic solution [66]. The thoracic paravertebral block is a potentially effective analgesic option in cases where TEA may not be practical or is contraindicated. Indications for analgesic paravertebral blocks include thoracic, unilateral breast surgery and open cholecystectomy, patients with multiple rib fractures, or when maintenance of hemodynamic stability is an important consideration.

For single-injection procedures, liposomal bupivacaine (Exparel) was approved by the Food and Drug Administration in 2011 for wound infiltration and has made its way into clinical practice. This long-acting formulation improves analgesia for painful procedures, such as hemorrhoidectomy [67] and bunionectomy [68], but its potential benefits in other types of surgery are still under study. Epidural administration of liposomal bupivacaine has been reported for analgesia after major abdominal procedures [69] and intra-articular injection of liposomal bupivacaine is currently being examined.

Finally, any clinical benefits derived from TEA clearly require administration of analgesic solution directly into the epidural space. When prospectively studied, TEA has a clinical failure rate that ranges from 16% to 23% or higher [57,70,71]. Causes of failure include technical insertion failure (up to 50% or more of cases) with dislodgement, ineffective analgesic solution, fat pedicle impingement, and incorrect intervertebral level of catheter relative to surgical incision accounting for the remainder [72–74]. Several insertion techniques are typically used, including loss of resistance (LOR) to air/saline, midline versus paramedian approach, and a hanging drop technique, but because no single technique has proved superior, the LOR technique using palpation of bony landmarks remains the most common and practical approach. After catheter insertion, 3 mL to 4 mL of concentrated local anesthetic solution (eg, 1.5% lidocaine with epinephrine) is typically injected to rule out intrathecal or intravascular positioning and to assess for dermatomal spread. This injection can be time consuming and associated with hemodynamic instability.

With such a high clinical failure rate of TEA, alternative approaches for epidural catheter insertion are gaining popularity. In ambulatory pain clinics, fluoroscopy has been routinely used for many years to identify the epidural space and confirm injection of epidurally administered medications. The use of fluoroscopy for confirmation of local anesthetic injection location could reasonably be extrapolated to thoracic epidural catheter placement. (In an analogous situation, use of brachial or lumbar plexus blocks for surgical anesthesia was limited by high failure rates until ultrasound guidance became widespread.) Fluoroscopic guidance can determine the exact location of the catheter tip and the associated characterization of injected fluid (dye) spread (cephalad/caudad, right/left) (Fig. 1). This approach eliminates the need for using dense local anesthetic solutions to confirm catheter placement. The authors have used this technique for the past 6 years [75] and recently

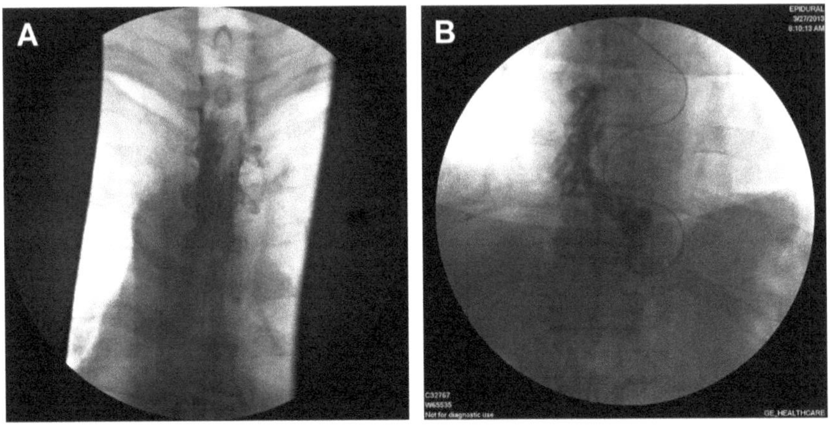

Fig. 1. After placement of a wire reinforced epidural catheter at the desired vertebral level, 2 mL of radiopaque dye is injected into the catheter to obtain an epidurogram. (*A*) The dye spread pattern is typical of an epidural location with bilateral symmetric spread along the spinal canal and some evidence of dye in the nerve root canals. (*B*) The catheter is clearly malpositioned outside of the epidural space.

completed a randomized, prospective clinical trial of 100 thoracotomy patients, examining the clinical impact of fluoroscopically guided catheter insertion compared with the traditional blind LOR approach. Fluoroscopic placement, using a wire reinforced epidural catheter (TheraCath, Arrow International, Reading, Pennsylvania) was associated with a significantly higher probability of correct catheter positioning and correctly positioned catheters were associated with shorter PACU and hospital length of stays (submitted for publication).

BENEFITS OF FLUOROSCOPIC GUIDANCE FOR PLACEMENT OF EPIDURAL CATHETERS

- Timely placement of catheters outside the operating room (OR). Catheters can be placed ahead of surgical start times avoiding delays in the OR. Average in-room to out-of-room time for catheter placement is 20 to 25 minutes.
- Eliminates the need for test doses of local anesthetic both before and after surgery—an epidurogram confirms placement in the epidural space and the absence of intrathecal or intravascular placement (see Fig. 1).
- Failure rate of catheters due to malposition, leakage, or dislodgement approaches zero.
- Precise, procedure-specific catheter placement minimizes epidural medication dosage and predicts postoperative functionality of the catheter [75].
- Patients can be more effectively sedated in the prone position used for fluoroscopy, which improves patient satisfaction.
- In a teaching environment, the immediate anatomic feedback during catheter placements has educational value.

More recently, the use of epidural waveform analysis (EWA), with pressure transduction through the needle, was examined as a confirmatory adjunct to conventional LOR. When the needle is correctly positioned in the epidural space, measurement of epidural pressure results in a pulsatile waveform. More recently, EWA-confirmed LOR and conventional LOR techniques were compared in a randomized controlled trial in patients undergoing thoracic or abdominal surgery and in patients with multiple rib fractures. Compared with conventional-LOR, EWA-confirmed LOR resulted in a lower rate of primary failure (2% vs 24%) [76]. This result is similar to what the authors observed using fluoroscopic guidance for placement of epidural catheters. The performance time was somewhat longer in the EWA-LOR group (11.2 minutes + 6.2 minutes vs 8.0 minutes + 4.6 minutes).

Considering that the primary failure rate of TEA remains high (especially in teaching centers [77]), incorporation of fluoroscopically guided or an EWA technique merits further investigation as a techniques to optimize the benefits and minimize the risks of TEA. In addition, even if additional studies confirm the benefits of increased primary success of TEA with these adjunctive confirmatory techniques, their practical, efficient, and cost-effective application in daily practice will require further investigation to justify more widespread use.

ANALGESIC SOLUTIONS

Most TEA protocols use dilute local anesthetic solutions (0.05%–0.1% bupivacaine or ropivacaine) to provide analgesia while preserving motor function. The addition of the lipophilic opioid fentanyl (eg, 2–4 μg/mL) provides better analgesia than local anesthetic alone without increased risk of respiratory depression [78]. Few studies have directly compared fentanyl to the more hydrophilic opioid, hydromorphone, as an analgesic adjunct to local anesthetics. One recent prospective, case-matched observational study demonstrated that epidural hydromorphone resulted in increased sedation compared with epidural fentanyl [79]. Randomized controlled studies directly comparing fentanyl to hydromorphone in equianalgesic concentrations are needed before any definitive conclusions can be made on the optimal opioid for use in conjunction with an epidurally administered local anesthetic solution. The rate and spread of the local anesthetic solution are additional, patient-specific components that may have an impact on the efficacy of TEA.

Epinephrine is a less commonly used analgesic adjunct for TEA. Randomized controlled trials have demonstrated, however, that epidural epinephrine (2 μg/mL) added to a bupivacaine-fentanyl solution increases sensory block spread, improves analgesia, and decreases serum fentanyl concentrations as well as decreasing sedation [80,81]. Infusion rates between 4 mL/h and 10 mL/h are commonly used and analgesia is improved when supplemented with PCEA. The PCEA approach offers patients an opportunity to self-administer additional local anesthetic (eg, 2–3 mL every 20 minutes) when they perceive suboptimal pain control.

THE PATIENT CARE TEAM

In larger hospitals, a dedicated APS, usually composed of physicians, nurses, and/or nurse practitioners (and physicians in training in teaching hospitals), improves TEA effectiveness and the patient experience [9]. When coupled with predetermined clinical pathways, this approach also shortens length of stay and lowers costs. Regardless of size, the key components of an effective APS include the following.

Consistency: development and maintenance of procedure-specific (and sometimes surgeon-specific) protocols for postoperative pain management
Efficiency: implementation of TEA with minimal time delays or impact on surgical schedules through improved institutional workflows
Efficacy: the postoperative analgesic plan is specifically designed to enhance the recovery profile of a specific procedure
Responsiveness: a system that adapts 24/7 to changes in surgical scheduling and patient status
Education: provider education regarding pain management creates a common language and solidifies goals surrounding optimal assessment and control of postoperative pain.

A dedicated nurse or nurse practitioner is invaluable for keeping the many components of an APS-based TEA service functioning and adapting to the constantly changing surgical environment [82]. When other providers are only intermittently involved with TEA patients, an APS nurse keeps the team on task and on time. Aside from ensuring the timely implementation of TEA protocols, the APS nurse may have other clinical tasks:

- Review the next day's surgical list to identify potential TEA candidates.
- Communicate with the surgical team to be sure all providers expect the same postoperative analgesia treatment plan.
- Review patient-specific data that can have an impact on TEA (eg, patient history, anticoagulation, laboratory tests, etc.) and plan ahead to avoid delays or last minute changes.
- Communicate with other hospital services involved (admitting staff, OR staff, postanesthesia care unit, floor, etc.) to ensure treatment plans are followed.
- Assist with epidural catheter placement (including patient care/sedation) organizing available personnel when multiple catheters need to be placed.
- See patients at key treatment points after surgery to ensure that analgesia is optimal. This may require multiple visits for some patients on a single day [82].

Essential components of the follow-up TEA patient visit

- Assessing quality of analgesia and adjusting epidural medications if necessary
- Suggesting use of supplemental analgesic medications when indicated
- Assessing for and managing side effects of TEA
- Optimizing patient recovery parameters, such as respiratory drive, effort (incentive spirometry), and ambulation

- Physically assessing integrity of epidural catheter dressing and insertion site
- Assisting with transition of patients from TEA to oral analgesics
- Communicating with physician and nursing staff regarding problems and changes in treatment plans

A critical component of effective TEA is ongoing education of patients and providers, which can be challenging in a busy hospital. An epidural teaching pamphlet given to a patient by the surgeon during a preadmission visit is an effective option. Without some preoperative patient education, information about the use of TEA often takes place at the bedside on the day of surgery when patients are least receptive to new information. For providers, basic epidural education should be provided to all nursing personnel before they begin work in a postsurgical unit. Most nurses also need to gain experience working with patients receiving TEA to become proficient at assessment and determination of a need for intervention. Timely and ongoing feedback/instruction by APS providers to hospital unit nurses is usually required to maintain high quality nursing assessments of patients with TEA.

Box 1: Sample monitoring protocol for patients with thoracic epidural analgesia

First 24 hours of new epidural

Continuous arterial oxygen saturation monitoring

Every 2 hours: respiratory status (depth, rate, regularity, and snoring), sedation scale (Pasero Opioid-Induced Sedation Scale if epidural contains an opioid)

Every 4 hours: vital signs and pain assessment

Every shift: motor and sensory examination[a] and dressing assessment

After 24 hours

Continuous arterial oxygen saturation monitoring

Every 4 hours: respiratory status (depth, rate regularity, and snoring), sedation scale, vital signs, and pain assessment

Every shift: motor and sensory examination and dressing assessment

[a] Sensory deficit: ask patient to point to numb and tingling skin areas (numbness and tingling at the incision site is common and usually normal). It is unexpected for a patient to have numbness or tingling of an extremity and this should be reported to APS. Motor deficit: ask patient to bend knees and lift buttocks off the mattress. Determine patient's ability to bear weight and ambulate. Most are able to do this without difficulty. All patients with an epidural are considered "at high risk to fall" and should not get out of bed without assistance. Notify the APS if the patient has new onset arm or leg weakness or inability to lift knees off bed or move legs.

Data from Pasero C, McCaffery M. Pain assessment and pharmacologic management. Elsevier; 2011.

NURSING ASSESSMENTS AND INTERVENTIONS FOR PATIENTS RECEIVING TEA (BOX 1)

- Patient excessively drowsy or sedated or a change in level of sedation
- Sensory deficit–numbness above axilla, numbness or tingling of extremities
- Motor deficit–new-onset arm or leg weakness, inability to lift knees off bed or move legs
- Any signs of local anesthetic toxicity: perioral numbness, ringing in ears, metallic taste, slow speech, irritability, twitching, seizures, cardiac dysrhythmias
- Protocol-based notification of APS prior to initiation of anticoagulation, including unfractionated heparin, warfarin, low-molecular-weight heparin, and antiplatelet agents, such as clopidogrel
- Management of catheter and dressing complications, such as disconnect, leaking fluid, or signs of inflammation at insertion site.
- Management of an epidural dressing that is not intact
- Inadequate analgesia

SUMMARY

TEA remains an effective and adaptable approach to not only managing postoperative pain but also providing a variety of other potential clinical benefits. There are multiple physiologic benefits of TEA making it perhaps the most widely tested modality for improving patient recovery after major surgery. Nonetheless, current anesthetic and surgical practices and the rapidly evolving nature of perioperative patient care mandate that decisions regarding use of TEA should be patient specific and undergo continuous re-evaluation.

References

[1] Crile G, Lower W. Anoci-Association. Philadelphia: Saunders; 1914.
[2] Tetzlaff J, Lautsenheiser F, Estafanous FG. Dr. George Crile-Early contributions to the theoretic basis for twenty-first century pain medicine. Reg Anesth Pain Med 2004;29(6):600–5.
[3] Cannon W. The wisdom of the body. New York: W.W. Norton & Company; 1932.
[4] Selye H. Role of the hypophysis in the pathogenesis of the diseases of adaption. Can Med Assoc J 1944;50:426–33.
[5] Griffiths D, Diamond A, Cameron J. Postoperative extradural analgesia following thoracic surgery: a feasibility study. Br J Anaesth 1975;48-55(47):1.
[6] Pflug A, Murphy T, Butler S, et al. The effects of postoperative peridural analgesia on pulmonary therapy and pulmonary complications. Anesthesiology 1974;41(1):8–17.
[7] Bromage P. Epidural analgesia. Philadelphia: WB Saunders Co; 1978.
[8] Coombs D, Danielson D, Pageau M, et al. Epidurally administered morphine for postcesarean analgesia. Surg Gynecol Obstet 1982;154(3):385–8.
[9] Werner M, Soholm L, Rotboll-Nielsen P, et al. Does an acute pain service improve postoperative outcome? Anesth Analg 2002;95:1361–72.
[10] Finks J, Osborne N, Birkmeyer J. Trends in hospital volume and operative mortality for high-risk surgery. N Engl J Med 2011;364(22):2128–37.
[11] Popping D, Elia N, Aken HV, et al. Impact of epidural analgesia on mortality and morbidity after surgery: systematic review and meta-analysis of randomized controlled trials. Ann Surg 2014;259(6):1056–67.
[12] Ballantyne J, Carr D, deFerranti S, et al. The comparative effects of postoperative analgesic therapies on pulmonary outcome: cumulative meta-analyses of randomized, controlled trials. Anesth Analg 1998;86:598–612.

[13] Popping D, Elia N, Marret E, et al. Protective effects of epidural analgesia on pulmonary complications after abdominal and thoracic surgery: a meta-analysis. Arch Surg 2008;143(10):990–9.
[14] Liu S, Carpenter R, Neal J. Epidural anesthesia and analgesia: their role in postoperative outcome. Anesthesiology 1995;82(6):1474–506.
[15] Liu S, Wu C. Effect of postoperative analgesia on major postoperative complications: a systematic update of the evidence. Anesth Analg 2007;104(3):689–702.
[16] Rodgers A, Walker N, Schug S, et al. Reduction of postoperative mortality and morbidity with epidural or spinal anaesthesia: results from overview of randomised trials. BMJ 2000;321:1493.
[17] Nishimori M, Low J, Zheng H, et al. Epidural pain relief versus systemic opioid-based pain relief for abdominal aortic surgery. Cochrane Database Syst Rev 2012;(7):CD00505.
[18] Park W, Thompson J, Lee K. Effect of epidural anesthesia and analgesia on perioperative outcome: a randomized, controlled Veterans Affairs Cooperative Study. Ann Surg 2001;234(4):560–71.
[19] Amini N, Kim Y, Hyder O, et al. A nationwide analysis of the use and outcomes of perioperative epidural analgesia in patients undergoing hepatic and pancreatic surgery. Am J Surg 2015;210:483–91.
[20] Lassen K, Coolsen M, Slim K, et al. Guidelines for perioperative care for pancreaticoduodenectomy: Enhanced Recovery After Surgery (ERAS) society recommendations. World J Surg 2013;37:240–58.
[21] Olausson K, Magnusdottir H, Lurje L, et al. Anit-ischemic and anti-anginal effects of thoracic epidural anesthesia versus those of conventional therapy in the treatment of severe refractory angina pectoris. Circulation 1997;96(7):2178–82.
[22] Breslow M, Jordan D, Christopherson R, et al. Epidural morphine decreases postoperative hypertension by attenuating sympathetic nervous system hyperactivity. JAMA 1989;261(24):3577–81.
[23] Beattie W, Badner N, Choi P. Epidural analgesia reduces postoperative myocardial infarction: a meta-analysis. Anesth Analg 2001;93:853–8.
[24] Fleisher L, Fleischmann K, Auerbach A, et al. 2014 ACC/AHA guideline on perioperative cardiovascular evaluation and management of patients undergoing noncardiac surgery. J Am Coll Cardiol 2014;64(22):e77–137.
[25] Liu S, Carpenter R, Mackey D, et al. Effects of perioperative analgesic technique on rate of recovery after colon surgery. Anesthesiology 1995;83(4):757–65.
[26] Ahn H, Bronge A, Ygge H, et al. Effects of continuous postoperative epidural analgesia on intestinal motility. Br J Surg 1988;75(12):1176–8.
[27] Jorgensen H, Wetterslev J, Moiniche S, et al. Epidural local anaesthetics versus opioid-based analgesic regimens on postoperative gastrointestinal paralysis, PONV and after abdominal surgery. Cochrane Database Syst Rev 2000;(4):CD001893.
[28] Scheinin B, Asantila R, Orko R. The effect of bupivacaine and morphine on pain and bowel function after colonic surgery. Acta Anaesthesiol Scand 1987;31:161–4.
[29] Jorgensen H, Fomsgaard J, Dirks J, et al. Effect of peri- an postoperative epidural anaesthesia on pain and gastrointestinal function after abdominal hysterectomy. Br J Anaesth 2001;87(4):577–83.
[30] Chou R, Gordon D, de Leon-Casasola O, et al. Management of postoperative pain: a clinical practice guideline from the American Pain Society, the American Society of Regional Anesthesia and Pain Medicine, and the American Society of Anesthesiologists' Committee on Regional Anesthesia, Executive Committee, and Administrative Council. J Pain 2016;17(2):131–57.
[31] Lattermann R, Schricker T, Wachter U, et al. Intraoperative epidural blockade prevents the increase in protein breakdown after abdominal surgery. Acta Anaesthesiol Scand 2001;45(9):1140–6.

[32] Usichenko T, Rottenbacher I, Kohlmann T, et al. Implementation of the quality management system improves postoperative pain treatment: a prospective pre-/post-interventional questionnaire study. Br J Anaesth 2013;110(1):87–95.
[33] Gustafsson U, Scott M, Schwenk W, et al. Guidelines for perioperative care in elective colonic surgery: Enhanced Recovery After Surgery (ERAS) Society Recommendations. World J Surg 2013;37:259–84.
[34] Miller T, Thacker J, White W, et al. Reduced length of hospital stay in colorectal surgery after implementation of an enhanced recovery protocol. Anesth Analg 2014;118(5):1052–61.
[35] Baldini G, Carli F. The Current and future role of regional anesthesia in enhanced recovery after surgery programs for abdominal surgery. Adv Anesth 2015;33:39–59.
[36] Nygren J, Thacker J, Carli F, et al. Guidelines for perioperative care in elective rectal/pelvic surgery: Enhanced Recovery After Surgery (ERAS) society recommendations. World J Surg 2013;37:285–305.
[37] Dahl J, Nielsen R, Wetterslev J, et al. Post-operative analgesic effects of paracetamol, NSAIDs, glucocorticoids, gabapentinoids and their combinations: a topical review. Acta Anaesthesiol Scand 2014;58(10):1165–81.
[38] Macario A, Royal M. A literature review of randomized clinical trials of intravenous acetaminophen (paracetamol) for acute postoperative pain. Pain Pract 2010;11(3):290–6.
[39] Apfel C, Turan A, Souza K, et al. Intravenous acetaminophen reduces postoperative nausea and vomiting: a systematic review and meta-analysis. Pain 2013;154(5):677–89.
[40] Duellman T, Gaffigan C, Milbrandt J, et al. Multi-modal, pre-emptive analgesia decreases the length of hospital stay following total joint arthroplasty. Orthopedics 2009;32(3):167.
[41] Kumar K, Kulkarni D, Gurajala I, et al. Pregabalin versus tramadol for postoperative pain management in patients undergoing lumbar laminectomy: a randomized, double-blinded, placebo-controlled study. J Pain Res 2013;24(6):471–8.
[42] Loftus R, Yeager M, Clark J, et al. Intraoperative ketamine reduces perioperative opiate consumption in opiate-dependent patients with chronic back pain undergoing back surgery. Anesthesiology 2010;113(3):639–46.
[43] Groudine S, Fisher H, Kaufman R, et al. Intravenous lidocaine speeds the return of bowel function, decreases postoperative pain, and shortens hospital stay in patients undergoing radical retropubic prostatectomy. Anesth Analg 1998;86:235–9.
[44] Carli F. Physiologic considerations of enhanced recovery after surgery (ERAS) programs: implications of the stress response. Can J Anaesth 2015;62(2):110–9.
[45] Yeager M, Colacchio T, Yu C, et al. Morphine inhibits spontaneous and cytokine-enhanced natural killer cell cytotoxcity in volunteers. Anesthesiology 1995;83(3):500–8.
[46] Horlocker T, Wedel D, Rowlingson J, et al. Regional anesthesia in the patient receiving antithrombotic or thrombolytic therapy. Reg Anesth Pain Med 2010;35(1):64–101.
[47] Cousins M, Wright C. Graft, muscle, skin blood flow after epidural block in vascular surgical procedures. Surg Gynecol Obstet 1971;133(1):59–64.
[48] Modig J, Borg T, Karlstrom G, et al. Thromboembolism after Total hip replacement: role of epidural and general anesthesia. Anesth Analg 1983;62:174–80.
[49] Christopherson R, Beattie C, Frank S, et al. Perioperative morbidity in patients randomized to epidural or general anesthesia for lower extremity vascular surgery. Anesthesiology 1993;79(3):422–34.
[50] Dodds T, Fillinger M, Walsh D, et al. Clinical outcomes after lower extremity revascularization: a comparison of epidural and general anesthesia. J Appl Res 2007;7(3):238–49.
[51] Rosenfeld B, Beattie C, Christopherson R, et al. The effects of different anesthetic regimens on fibrinolysis and the development of postoperative arterial thrombosis. Anesthesiology 1993;79(3):435–43.
[52] Tuman K, McCarthy R, March R, et al. Effects of epidural anesthesia and analgesia on coagulation and outcome after major vascular surgery. Anesth Analg 1991;73:696–704.
[53] Andreae M, Andreae D. Regional anaesthesia to prevent chronic pain after surgery: a Cochrane systematic review and meta-analysis. Br J Anaesth 2013;111(5):711–20.

[54] Zaouter C, Pepa K, Carli F. Less urinary tract infection by earlier removal of bladder catheter in surgical patients receiving thoracic epidural analgesia. Reg Anesth Pain Med 2009;34(6):542–8.
[55] Basse L, Werner M, Kehlet H. Is urinary drainage necessary during continuous epidural analgesia after colonic resection? Reg Anesth Pain Med 2000;25(5):498–501.
[56] Wu C, Benson A, Hobson D, et al. Initiating an enhanced recovery pathway program: an anesthesiology department's perspective. Jt Comm J Qual Patient Saf 2015;41(10): 447–56.
[57] Sugimoto M, Nesbit L, Barton J, et al. Epidural anesthesia dysfunction is associated with postoperative complications after pancreatectomy. J Hepatobiliary Pancreat Sci 2016;23(2):102–9.
[58] Rosero E, Joshi G. Nationwide incidence of serious complications of epidural analgesia in the United States. Acta Anaesthesiol Scand 2016;60:810–20.
[59] Horlocker T, Burton A, Connis R, et al. Practice guidelines for the prevention, detection, and management of respiratory depression associated with neuraxial opiod administration: an updated report by the American Society of Anesthesiologists Task Force on Neuraxial Opiods and the American Society of Regional Anesthesia and Pain Medicine. Anesthesiology 2016;123(3):535–52.
[60] Williams-Russo P, Sharrock N, Mattis S, et al. Cognitive effects after epidural vs general anesthesia in older adults: a randomized trial. JAMA 1995;274(1):44–50.
[61] Steinbrook R. Epidural anesthesia and gastrointestinal motility. Anesth Analg 1998;86: 837–44.
[62] Rafi A. Abdominal field block: a new approach via the lumbar triangle. Anaesthesia 2001;56(10):1024–6.
[63] Hebbard P, Fugiwara Y, Shibata Y, et al. Ultrasound-guided transversus abdominis plane (TAP) block. Anaesth Intensive Care 2007;35(4):616–7.
[64] Hebbard P. Subcostal transversus abdominis plane block under ultrasound guidance. Anesth Analg 2008;106(2):674–5.
[65] Eason M, Wyatt R. Paravertebral thoracic block - a reappraisal. Anesth Analg 1979;106(2):674–5.
[66] Cheema S, Ilsley D, Richardson J, et al. A thermographic study of paravertebral analgesia. Anaesthesia 1995;50:118–21.
[67] Gorfine S, Onel E, Patou G, et al. Bupivacaine extended-release liposome injection for prolonged postsurgical analgesia in patients undergoing hemorrhoidectomy: a multicenter, randomized, double-blind, placebo-controlled trial. Dis Colon Rectum 2011;54(12): 1552–9.
[68] Golf M, Daniels S, Onel E. A phase 3, randomized, placebo controlled trial of DepoFoam bupivacaine (extended-release bupivacaine local analgesic) in bunionectomy. Adv Ther 2011;28(9):776–88.
[69] Boogaerts J, Lafont N, Declercq A, et al. Epidural administration of liposome-associated bupivacaine for the management of postsurgical pain: a first study. J Clin Anesth 1994;6: 315–20.
[70] Burstal R, Wegener F, Hayes C, et al. Epidural analgesia: prospective audit of 1062 patients. Anaesth Intensive Care 1998;26(2):165–72.
[71] McLeod G, Davies H, Munnoch N, et al. Postoperative pain relief using thoracic epidural analgesia: outstanding success and disappointing failures. Anaesthesia 2001;56(1):75–81.
[72] Hermanides J, Hollmann M, Stevens M, et al. Failed epidural: causes and management. Br J Anaesth 2012;109:144–54.
[73] Pan P, Bogard T, Owen M. Incidence and characteristics of failures in obstetric neuraxial analgesia and anesthesia: a retrospective analysis of 19, 259 deliveries. Int J Obstet Anesth 2004;13:227–33.
[74] Collier C. Why obstetric epidurals fail: a study of epidurograms. Int J Obstet Anesth 1996;5: 19–31.

[75] Yeager M, Bae E, Parra M, et al. Fluorsocopically-assisted epidural catheter placement: an exploratory analysis of 303 pre-operative epidurograms. Acta Anaesthesiol 2016;60(4): 513–9.
[76] Arnuntasupakul V, Zundert TV, Vijitpavan A, et al. A randomized comparison between conventional and waveform-confirmed loss of resistance for thoracic epidural blocks. Reg Anesth Pain Med 2016;41(3):368–73.
[77] Tran QD, Zundert TV, Aliste J, et al. Primary failure of thoracic epidural analgesia in training centers. Reg Anesth Pain Med 2016;41(3):309–13.
[78] De Leon-Casasola O, Parker B, Lema M, et al. Postoperative epidural bupivacaine-morphine therapy. Experience with 4,227 surgical cancer patients. Anesthesiology 1994;81: 368–75.
[79] Nguyen M, Zimmerman L, Meloche K, et al. Hydromorphone vs fentanyl for epidural analgesia and anesthesia. Am J Surg 2016;211(3):565–70.
[80] Niemi G, Breivik H. Epinephrine markedly improves thoracic epidural analgesia produced by a small-dose infusion of ropivacaine, fentanyl, and epinephrine after major throacic or abdominal surgery: a randomized, double-blinded crossover study with and without epinephrine. Anesth Analg 2002;94(6):1598–605.
[81] Curatolo M. Is epinephrine unfairly neglected for postoperative mixtures? Anesth Analg 2002;94(6):1381–3.
[82] Pasero C, McCaffery M. Pain assessment and pharmacologic management. St. Louis (MO): Elsevier; 2011.

Advances in Anesthesia 34 (2016) 161–180

ADVANCES IN ANESTHESIA

Evidence-Based Perioperative Management of Cardiac Medications in Patients Presenting for Noncardiac Surgery

Jeremy M. Bennett, MD*, Kara Siegrist, MD

Division of Cardiothoracic Anesthesiology, Vanderbilt University Medical Center, 1215 21st Avenue South, 5160F Medical Center East North Tower, Nashville, TN 37232, USA

Keywords

• Beta-blockers • Angiotensin-converting enzyme inhibitors
• Angiotensin receptor blockers • Alpha-2 receptor blockers • Anticoagulants
• Antiplatelet agents • HMG CoA reductase inhibitors/statins
• Cardiovascular disease

Key points

- Cardiovascular disease is a major cause of morbidity and mortality not only in the United States but throughout the world.
- Many classes of pharmacologic agents are utilized in the treatment of cardiovascular disease.
- New agents are constantly being introduced into practice. It is important for the anesthesiologist to be familiar with their mechanism of action and guidelines for use.

INTRODUCTION

Cardiovascular disease is the leading cause of death in the United States and is on pace to become the leading cause in the world. According to the Centers for Disease Control and Prevention, in 2014, 610,000 people died of heart disease in the United States [1]. Coronary artery disease (CAD) is the most prevalent subset of cardiovascular disease. CAD leads to major morbidity with more than 735,000 Americans affected by myocardial infarctions each year [2]. With the increase in prevalence of cardiovascular disease and expected continued growth of the diseased population, health care providers must be

The authors have no conflicts of interest or financial engagements to disclose.

*Corresponding author. *E-mail address:* jeremy.m.bennett@vanderbilt.edu

http://dx.doi.org/10.1016/j.aan.2016.07.010

knowledgeable regarding drug therapies and ongoing advancements in therapies used to treat these patients [3].

Confusion often exists regarding appropriate management of cardiovascular-based medications for patients presenting for noncardiac surgery. Specific concerns revolve around need to continue or discontinue medications; the timing of discontinuation before, as well as following, surgery; and the benefits of initiating medications in patients previously naïve to those drugs. This article summarizes the pharmacology of commonly encountered cardiovascular medications, the indications for therapy, and most recent evidence-based guidelines from the American College of Cardiology/American Heart Association (ACC/AHA) regarding appropriate management in patients who are scheduled for noncardiac surgery.

Recommendations are given level of benefit and level of evidence designations based on the most recent 2014 ACC/AHA guidelines. Table 1 presents recommendation and evidence designations to aid familiarity with the perioperative recommendations provided.

Statin therapy

Pharmacology

HMG-CoA reductase inhibitors are generically known as statins owing to the common ending of each drug's generic name. These drugs include simvastatin (Zocor), atorvastatin (Lipitor), pravastatin (Pravachol), and rosuvastatin (Crestor), in addition to others that are not available in the United States. These drugs are currently considered first-line agents in the management of elevated cholesterol and hyperlipidemia in patients at risk for cardiovascular disease [4]. 3-Hydroxy-3-methylglutaryl coenzyme A reductase inhibitor (HMG-CoA) reductase is the rate-limiting enzyme involved in the synthesis of cholesterol though the mevalonic acid pathway (Fig. 1). Inhibiting this enzyme reduces blood cholesterol levels more than diet modification alone. Inhibition of HMG-CoA reductase results in upregulation of the low-density lipoprotein (LDL) receptor within the liver, which results in increased degradation of blood LDL. This subsequently lowers cholesterol while resulting in modest increases in high-density lipoprotein (HDL) [5].

Table 1
Class of recommendation and level of evidence for guidelines

Class of Recommendation	
I	Intervention is useful and effective
IIa	Intervention likely useful and effective based on weight of evidence
IIb	Intervention potentially useful and effective based on evidence or opinion
III	Intervention is not helpful and possibly harmful
Level of evidence	
A	Several RCTs; strong experimental findings
B	Limited evidence from observational trials or a single RCT
C	Expert opinion or standard of care; case reports or series

Abbreviation: RCT, randomized controlled trial.

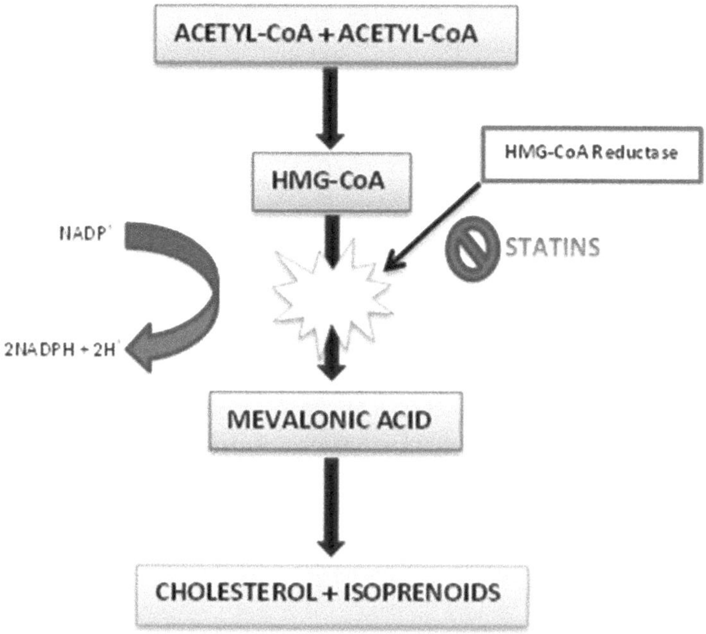

Fig. 1. HMG-CoA reductase inhibition of cholesterol synthesis. NADP, nicotinamide adenine dinucleotide phosphate.

Statins have a generally favorable safety profile and are well tolerated by most patients with specific treatment goals aimed at adjustment of LDL, HDL, and total cholesterol levels. Myalgia, manifesting as muscle pain or soreness occurs in some patients with a small portion developing life-threatening rhabdomyolysis. This myalgia is also known as statin-induced myopathy and the mechanism is poorly understood but may be related to decreases in downstream metabolites of the mevalonic acid pathway beyond cholesterol that have effects in skeletal muscle [6]. Patients who experience statin-induced myopathy experience decreased compliance, have reduced exercise tolerance, are at risk for life-threatening rhabdomyolysis, and will usually have this form of cholesterol therapy discontinued.

Indications for therapy
HMG-CoA reductase inhibitors are first-line therapy for management of hypercholesterolemia. Additional therapeutic efficacy includes hypertriglyceridemia, hyperlipidemia, atherosclerosis, familial hypercholesterolemia, and stroke prevention.

Perioperative statin recommendations
Class I, B. Perioperative continuation of statins in patients who are already prescribed statin therapy is advisable.

Class IIa, B. Initiation of statin therapy in patients not previously prescribed statins who present for vascular surgery is reasonable.

Class IIb, C. Perioperative initiation of statin therapy in patients not previously prescribed statins and who present for noncardiac, nonvascular surgery may be considered in patients with elevated cardiac risk factors.

Recent ACC/AHA guidelines on perioperative management of statin therapy indicate that continuation of statins in patients already prescribed therapy is advisable [7]. A retrospective study involving 329 hospitals in the United States demonstrated a decrease in all-cause mortality in major, noncardiac surgery when patients either continued or had statin therapy initiated in the first 2 hospital days. This reduction in mortality remained after propensity matching was performed [8]. In a large, retrospective study of patients undergoing intermediate risk, nonvascular, noncardiac surgery, patients previously taking statin therapy had a 30 day mortality of 4 out of 274 (1.45%) versus 31 out of 478 (6.48%) for patients not previously on statins ($P<.002$) [9]. After propensity matching, the decrease in 30 day mortality was still evident in patients on statins.

Initiation of statin therapy in the perioperative period in previously naïve patients is reasonable in vascular surgery. A meta-analysis of studies including 4 randomized controlled trials and 20 observational trials demonstrated improvement in primary study outcomes in which subjects were either continued on statin therapy or were randomized to initiate statin therapy [10]. Furthermore, in patients presenting for noncardiac surgery there does not seem to be a detriment for initiation of statin therapy if patients have at least 1 risk factor for cardiovascular disease. This recommendation, although given class IIB strength in the most recent ACC/AHA guidelines, likely comes from ambiguous timing of statin therapy in several observational trials. It is not well delineated if patients presented with previously prescribed statin therapy or had statins begun shortly before or on the day of surgery. In cardiac surgery there has been increasing concern for acute kidney injury following initiation of statin in naïve patients [11]; however, because this has not yet been demonstrated in noncardiac surgery, it is reasonably safe to start therapy based on current evidence.

Based on the most recent guidelines statin therapy should not be discontinued before noncardiac surgery. If statin therapy was held before surgery it is advisable to resume therapy as soon as possible to reduce the incidence of cardiovascular events and mortality in the postoperative period.

Angiotensin-converting enzyme inhibitors or angiotensin receptor blockers

Pharmacology

Angiotensin-converting enzyme (ACE)-inhibitors and angiotensin receptor blockers (ARBs) are primarily used for the treatment of hypertension, as well as congestive heart failure, and will be reviewed together due to similar profiles as well as therapeutic efficacy. Several types of ACE inhibitors are available for outpatient treatment, including benazepril (Lotensin), captopril

(Capoten), enalapril (Vasotec), fosinopril (Monopril), lisinopril (Prinivil, Zestril), quinapril (Accupril), Ramipril (Altace), trandolapril (Mavik), and others not commonly encountered or available. Enalaprilat is an intravenous form of ACE inhibitor that is frequently used in the perioperative period when patients are unable to take oral medications. ACE inhibitors are commonly identified by their common generic name ending "-pril." ARBs include: candesartan (Atacand), irbesartan (Avapro), losartan (Cozaar), olmesartan (Benicar), telmisartan (Micardis), and valsartan (Diovan). ARBs are recognized the common generic name ending"-sartan."

The mechanism of action of ACE inhibitors or ARBs relates to their effect on the renin-angiotensin-aldosterone-system [12]. Renin is stimulated for release within the juxtaglomerular apparatus of the kidney during periods of hypotension, decrement in serum sodium concentration, and sympathetic stimulation via beta receptors. Once released, renin cleaves amino acids from angiotensinogen, a preprotein produced in the liver. This enzymatic cleavage creates angiotensin I, which circulates in the blood to the lungs, where ACE cleaves additional amino acids from angiotensin I, forming angiotensin II. This protein has powerful constrictive properties on the vasculature, as well as a role in salt and water absorption from the kidney. ACE inhibitors work to prevent the conversion of angiotensin I to angiotensin II within the pulmonary system.

Angiotensin II normally acts on the body by increasing blood pressure through receptors on the vascular endothelium, as well as by increasing salt and water balance via release of aldosterone. Ventricular remodeling occurs due to promotion of proto-oncogenes, which results in hypertrophy and fibrosis of myocardial tissue. Vasopressin (antidiuretic hormone [ADH]) is released by the posterior pituitary to further increase water retention by the renal system. ACE inhibitors reduce these effects by limiting the production of angiotensin II. ARBs work by reducing the effectiveness of angiotensin II binding to smooth muscle receptors in the vascular endothelium, thus reducing vasoconstriction. ARBs additionally reduce release of vasopressin (ADH), as well as aldosterone. Furthermore, vasopressin has direct vasoconstrictive effects in the systemic circulation via the V1a receptor and reduced release results in further decreases in arteriolar resistance.

Indications for therapy

Angiotensin receptor blocking medications are used primarily for hypertensive therapy but have received continued indications for congestive heart failure, cerebrovascular accident prevention, and recent myocardial infarction.

Current guidelines and recommendations

Class IIa, B. Continuation of ACE inhibitors or ARBs is reasonable before noncardiac surgery.

Class IIa, C. If ACE inhibitors or ARBs are held before noncardiac surgery, it is reasonable to resume therapy as soon as is clinically possible.

ACE inhibitors and ARBs are heavily prescribed medications due to their beneficial effects on arterial blood pressure, reducing cardiovascular risk, beneficial effects in congestive heart failure, and adjustment in cardiac remodeling [12,13]. Side effects from ACE inhibitors, often attributable to elevated bradykinin levels, can reduce patient compliance and may require cessation due to concern for life-threatening angioedema. One of the most common side effects of ACE inhibitors is a dry, persistent cough, which frequently necessitates adjustment of the medication or a change to an ARB. Although largely prescribed, available clinical trials are mostly observational or small, limiting evaluation of potential benefits versus risks, particularly in the surgical setting.

One of the biggest concerns related to ACE inhibitors and ARBs is the concern for perioperative hypotension with anecdotal reports of refractory hypotension to standard vasopressor therapy. The decision to hold therapy the day before surgery has been an ongoing question because studies evaluating angiotensin blockade in the perioperative periods have not been large enough or definitive to come to any absolute conclusion. An observational trial evaluating 267 subjects with hypertension and prescribed ACE inhibitors or ARBs demonstrated a significantly increased incidence of hypotension for up to 30 minutes after induction of general anesthesia (odds ratio [OR] 1.74, $P = .02$) [14]. Hypotension occurred in subjects having taken an ACE inhibitor or ARB up to 10 hours before surgery compared with those who held their medication for more than 10 hours. A retrospective study evaluating effects of angiotensin blockade on respiratory complications in 76,525 subjects did not find any worsened pulmonary outcomes in patients taking ACE inhibitors. A secondary endpoint of hypotension was not seen in subjects treated with ACE inhibitor (OR 0.98, $P = .54$) [15]. Although the investigators did not find a significant difference in hypotension between the groups, there was an increased use of vasopressors in subjects treated with ACE inhibitors.

A prospective, observational study of 17,758 subjects demonstrated no difference in intraoperative hypotension in subjects on chronic ACE inhibitors or ARBs versus propensity-matched controls except in subjects who took a concomitant diuretic the day of surgery [16]. Subjects on beta-blockers, calcium channel blockers (CCBs), or combinations with diuretics and ACE inhibitors did not, however, demonstrate significant intraoperative hypotension as may be expected. Furthermore, despite the findings in subjects on diuretics and ACE inhibitors or ARBs, an increase in postoperative morbidity or mortality was not seen between the groups. A meta-analysis of clinical studies demonstrated an increase in intraoperative hypotension following induction of general anesthesia in subjects who took their ACE inhibitor or ARB on the day of surgery without an increase in morbidity or mortality between the study patients [17].

Although some studies have not demonstrated an association, intraoperative hypotension following induction of general anesthesia does seem to occur more frequently in patients taking ACE inhibitors or ARBs before surgery. Patients taking them the night before a morning operation may still be at risk. However, despite the incidence of hypotension and increased use of vasopressors, worsened outcomes have not been demonstrated. Furthermore, there is concern that patients who have their medication held before surgery may be less likely to resume this once discharged from the hospital. Surgical patient data are lacking in this regard but evidence of medication compliance, particularly in patients with heart failure or prior myocardial infarction, has been shown to reduce readmission rates for comorbid conditions [18]. Vasopressin or analogs may be beneficial in counteracting angiotensin inhibitor–induced hypotension; however, caution should be taken due to concerns for reduced mesenteric blood flow [19].

Based on these studies and recent perioperative guidelines [7], continuation of ACE inhibitors or ARBs is reasonable in the perioperative period. If significant enough concern exists for patient intolerance with hypotension of any amount (eg, carotid endarterectomy, aortic stenosis), then withholding ACE inhibitors or ARBs before surgery is acceptable. If therapy is held, there should be a plan in place to resume medications as soon as is reasonably possible.

Alpha-2 agonists

Pharmacology

Alpha-2 agonists act on the sympathetic nervous system, resulting in antihypertensive effects and sedation. Clonidine (Catapres, Duraclon, Kapvay) is among the most commonly used alpha-2 agonists. Other drugs that act on the alpha-2 receptor include mivazerol, guanfacine (Ituniv, Tenex), tizanidine (Zanaflex), and methyldopa. Dexmedetomidine (Precedex) is not discussed in this article because it is not an outpatient medication.

Alpha-2 agonists bind the alpha-2 receptor on endothelium and in the central nervous system. Alpha-2 receptors are Gi protein-coupled receptors that reduce cyclic adenosine monophosphate (cAMP) within the cell. The net result in the peripheral vasculature is decreased smooth muscle contraction and vasodilation. In the central nervous system, sedation often predominates.

Indications for therapy

Antihypertensive therapy, sedation, treatment of attention-deficit/hyperactivity disorder.

Current guidelines and recommendations

Class III, B. Alpha-2 agonists are not recommended to prevent cardiac complications in the perioperative period.

Alpha-2 agonists are used to manage arterial blood pressure. Clonidine is the most commonly encountered alpha-2 agonist and is the main focus of studies and recommendations. A randomized, double-blinded clinical trial of 190 subjects (clonidine, n = 125 vs placebo, n = 65) in 2004 demonstrated improved (ie, decreased) myocardial ischemia and reduced mortality for up to 2 years following surgery [20]. Several additional small studies (<300 subjects per trial) also demonstrated improved myocardial outcomes with minimal hemodynamic disturbances. Based on this evidence, clonidine initiation and perioperative continuation through the perioperative period was embraced as a cardiac protective measure. More recent studies, however, have not demonstrated the cardioprotective effect and have instead demonstrated significant hypotension associated with initiation or continuation of clonidine.

Evaluation of effects on acute kidney injury in patients receiving clonidine and aspirin demonstrated increased risk for hypotension with resultant kidney injury [21]. The PeriOperative Ischemic Evaluation (POISE)-2 trial, a robust, multicenter, and multinational study, evaluated the effects of aspirin and clonidine using a 2-by-2 factorial trial design in 10,010 subjects at risk for vascular complications undergoing noncardiac surgery. Subjects were placed into 1 of 4 groups: aspirin with clonidine placebo, aspirin with clonidine, aspirin placebo with clonidine, and aspirin placebo with clonidine placebo [22]. Clonidine did not significantly reduce the primary outcome of mortality or nonfatal myocardial infarction. Moreover, more subjects in the clonidine group experienced nonfatal cardiac arrest (16 subjects vs 5 subjects; hazard ratio [HR] 3.20, 95% CI, 1.17–8.73, $P = .02$), with pulseless electrical activity and asystole seen in 85% of those. Furthermore, although there was no difference between hospital or intensive care length of stay, clinically significant hypotension (2385 subjects vs 1854 subjects; HR 1.32, CI 1.24–1.4, $P < .001$) and bradycardia (600 subjects vs 403 subjects; HR 1.49, CI 1.32–1.69; $P < .001$) were observed more in subjects receiving clonidine versus placebo.

Based on the results of more recent trials, including the robust POISE-2 trial, perioperative administration or continuation of previously prescribed clonidine is not recommended to prevent myocardial ischemia or other cardiovascular complications (class III, level of evidence B). For patients on long-term clonidine administration, however, it is wise to monitor for potential rebound hypertension, which may be severe in some cases, and resume their antihypertensive medication as soon as possible (class III, level of evidence C).

Beta-blockers

Overview and pharmacology

For many years, beta-blocker therapy was considered the first-line agent in the treatment of primary hypertension. However, beta-blocker therapy has come under scrutiny with the advent of different classes of antihypertensives, such as CCBs, ACE-inhibitors, and ARBs. As of 2007, The AHA no longer recommends beta-blockers as first-line therapy for primary hypertension [23]. Currently, beta-blocker therapy is advised as a second-line therapy to CCB, ACE inhibitors, or ARBs for hypertension treatment due to its proven inferiority to other agents in reducing stroke, cardiovascular mortality, and all-cause mortality [24].

The pharmacologic class of beta-blockers is wide and varying in many characteristics, such as beta-receptor selectivity, half-life, lipid solubility, and additional pharmacologic mechanisms (eg, vasodilation, alpha receptor selectivity). In general, beta-blockers are thought to reduce blood pressure via a reduction in cardiac output via beta-receptor inhibition. Other proposed mechanisms include beta-1 mediated inhibition at the juxtaglomerular apparatus, causing a decrease in renin release, increased vascular compliance causing reductions in venous return, and decreased norepinephrine release [25]. Newer agents, such as carvedilol (Coreg) and nebivolol (Bystolic), have additional mechanisms for blood pressure reduction via alpha-receptor inhibition and nitric oxide–medicated vasodilation, respectively [24]. Table 2 contains an abbreviated list of commonly used beta-blockers and their respective pharmacologic properties.

Indications for therapy

Beta-blocker pharmacotherapy is approved as second-line antihypertensive therapy, often in addition to another pharmacologic class of antihypertensives, such as CCBs, ACE-inhibitors, ARBs, and others. Beta-blocker therapy is also

Table 2
Pharmacology of beta-blockers

	Receptor selectivity	Route	Half-life (h)	Metabolism	Special Considerations
Atenolol (Tenormin)	Beta-1	po	6–7	Renal	
Bisoprolol (Zebeta)	Beta-1	po	9–12	Renal	
Carvedilol (Coreg)	Beta-1, Beta-2	po	7–10	Hepatic	Alpha-1 blockade
Esmolol (Brevibloc)	Beta-1	IV	8–10 min	Enzymatic	Plasma-esterase degradation
Labetalol (Trandate)	Beta-1, Beta-2, alpha-1	po, IV	6–8 (PO) 5–6 (IV)	Hepatic	3:1 B > a (po); 7:1 B > a (IV)
Metoprolol (Lopressor, Toprol)	Beta-1	po, IV	Tartrate: 3–4 Succinate: 3–7	Hepatic	
Nebivolol (Bystolic)	Beta-1	po	11–30	Hepatic	Nitric oxide–mediated vasodilation; B3 Receptor agonist
Propranolol (Inderal)	Beta-1, Beta-2	po	3.5–6	Hepatic	
Sotalol (Betapace)	Beta-1, Beta-2	po	12	Renal excretion	Class III antiarrhythmic properties (K channel blocker)

Abbreviation: IV, intavenous.

Adapted from Benowitz NL. Antihypertensive agents. Basic and clinical pharmacology. 12th edition. McGraw-Hill; 2012. Chapter 11.

indicated in the treatment of chronic stable angina and atrial arrhythmias. Propranolol is also indicated for migraine prophylaxis and bleeding esophageal varices prevention. Carvedilol is indicated in treatment of heart failure for all ranges of severity and in treatment of decreased left ventricular function post-myocardial infarction. Metoprolol has also been used in stable symptomatic heart failure.

Current guidelines and recommendations
Class I B. Beta-blockers should be continued in patients undergoing surgery who have been on beta-blockers chronically.

Class I B. Control of the ventricular rate using a beta-blocker or nondihydropyridine calcium channel antagonist is recommended for patients with paroxysmal, persistent, or permanent atrial fibrillation.

Class IIa. A heart rate control (resting rate <80 beats per minute) strategy is reasonable for symptomatic management of atrial fibrillation.

Class IIb C. In patients with intermediate or high-risk myocardial ischemia noted in preoperative risk stratification tests, it may be reasonable to begin perioperative beta-blockers.

Class IIb B. In patients with 3 or more revised cardiac risk factors (diabetes mellitus, heart failure, CAD, renal insufficiency, cerebrovascular accident), it may be reasonable to begin beta-blockers before surgery.

Class IIb B. In patients with a compelling long-term indication for beta-blocker therapy but no other revised cardiac risk factors, initiating beta-blockers in the perioperative setting as an approach to reduce perioperative risk is of uncertain benefit.

Class III B. Beta-blocker therapy should not be started on the day of surgery.

Perhaps the most influential study regarding perioperative beta-blocker therapy was the POISE trial published in 2008, now known as POISE-1. The POISE-1 trial included more than 8000 subjects undergoing noncardiac surgery randomized to initiate extended release metoprolol or placebo 2 to 4 hours preoperatively, which was then continued for 30 days postoperatively. The results of the POISE-1 trial demonstrated that perioperative extended-release metoprolol reduced the risk of myocardial infarction, need for cardiac revascularization, and atrial fibrillation within 30 days postoperatively. However, there was an increased risk of death (relative risk 1.29), stroke, hypotension, and bradycardia in subjects having received beta-blocker therapy [26].

According to the 2014 Clinical Practice Guidelines set forth by the ACC/AHA, there is insufficient evidence to recommend starting a beta-blocker in noncardiac surgical patients within 1 day of surgery due to the increased risk of stroke, hypotension, bradycardia, and death [27].

Guidelines do support continuing beta-blocker therapy in patients already receiving long-term treatment preoperatively for noncardiac surgery patients. Initiation of beta-blocker therapy should be considered in patients with 3 or more cardiovascular risk factors or if preoperative testing indicative of ischemia (eg, positive stress test) is discovered. Therapy should be started several days before surgery with titration of dose to a goal heart rate of 60 to 70 beats per minute [27,28].

Antiplatelet agents

Overview and pharmacology

During acute coronary events, the fibrous cap containing atheromatous plaque ruptures, exposing prothrombotic substances that are released into the endothelium, leading to formation of a thrombus [29]. Prevention of clot formation or expansion of thrombus can prevent complete and total occlusion of the vascular lumen. Platelet activation and adhesion plays a major role in thrombus formation at the site of vascular injury. Fig. 2 demonstrates the multitude of platelet activation receptors and the pharmacologic agents that block these mechanisms of activation.

Aspirin is an irreversible, nonspecific cyclooxygenase (COX) inhibitor that inhibits synthesis of thromboxane A2, a potent prostaglandin that leads to platelet degranulation and aggregation. Aspirin has a 170-fold higher affinity for COX-1 than COX-2 and irreversibly inhibits COX-1 enzyme, inhibiting thromboxane production for the lifespan of a platelet (7–10 days). Peak plasma levels (and thus platelet inhibition) occur 30 minutes after oral administration for nonenteric-coated aspirin and 3 to 4 hours after administration for enteric-coated aspirin. Aspirin's antiplatelet effect is dose-dependent [30]. Factors affecting return of functional platelet aggregation after cessation of aspirin include the dose of aspirin, rate of platelet turnover, time from discontinuation, and patient-specific factors. In general, it is safe to assume that after 10 days of

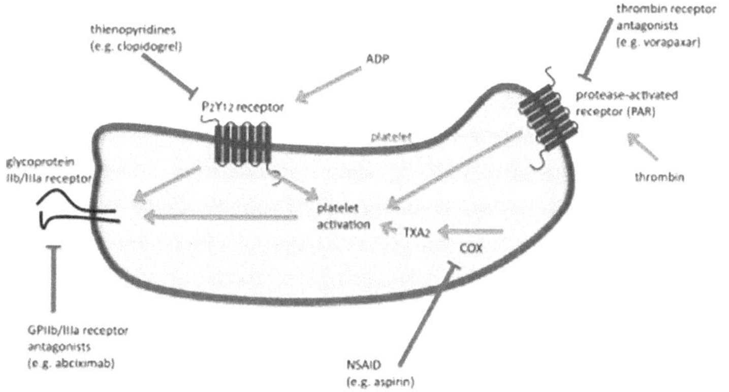

Fig. 2. Inhibition of platelet activation via pharmacologic antagonism.

aspirin discontinuation, 100% of the platelet pool would have turned over with normal resumption of COX enzyme activity [31].

Nonaspirin nonsteroidal anti-inflammatory drugs (NSAIDs) (eg, ibuprofen, naproxen, indomethacin, diclofenac) also inhibit COX but in a reversible and competitive fashion. A subclass of NSAIDs has been termed COX-2 selective and includes drugs such as meloxicam, etodolac, celecoxib, and nabumetone; however, these drugs still exhibit some COX-1 inhibition but do not alter platelet function to a clinically significant degree.

The phosphodiesterase inhibitors (PDEs) are another class of antiplatelet therapy. Dipyridamole and cilostazol are the most commonly encountered drugs in this class. PDE inhibitors act on cAMP and cyclic guanosine monophosphate (cGMP) to affect their antiplatelet action. The platelet surface expresses 3 PDE receptors, PDE-2, 3, and 5. Dipyridamole acts on PDE3 and PDE-5, increasing cAMP and cGMP levels, and causing reduced platelet aggregation and vasodilation. Dipyridamole is often used together with aspirin for synergistic antiplatelet effects. Cilostazol inhibits PDE-3 and also has arterial vasodilator activity, thus causing inhibition of vasoconstriction and platelet aggregation (secondary effect) [31].

The thienopyridine class of antiplatelet agents includes drugs such as ticlopidine (Ticlid), clopidogrel (Plavix), and prasugrel (Effient). Thienopyridines work via irreversible inhibition of the P2Y12 (adenosine diphosphate) ADP receptor mediated platelet aggregation. Platelet glycoprotein IIb/IIIa receptor inhibitors block activation of the platelet by fibrinogen, fibronectin, and von Willebrand factor. Glycoprotein IIb/IIIa activation is in the final steps of the platelet aggregation cascade. Examples of drugs in this class include abciximab (ReoPro), eptifibatide (Integrilin), and tirofiban (Aggrastat).

New antiplatelet agents are being unveiled at a rapid rate. Ticagrelor (Brilinta) is a reversible P2Y12 ADP receptor inhibitor approved for acute coronary syndrome (ACS) when used in conjunct with aspirin. The recent Platelet Inhibition and Patient Outcomes (PLATO) trial demonstrated superiority of ticagrelor over clopidogrel when used in ACS versus endpoints of cardiovascular death and stroke; however, it did increase surgical bleeding [32].

Current guidelines and recommendations

Class I C. In patients undergoing urgent noncardiac surgery during the first 4 to 6 weeks after bare metal stent or drug eluting stent (DES) implantation, dual antiplatelet therapy (DAPT) should be continued unless the relative risk of bleeding outweighs the benefit of the prevention of stent thrombosis.

Class I C. In patients who have received coronary stents and must undergo surgical procedures that mandate the discontinuation of P2Y12 platelet receptor inhibitor therapy, it is recommended that aspirin be continued if possible and the P2Y12 platelet receptor inhibitor be restarted as soon as possible after surgery.

Class I C. Management of the perioperative antiplatelet therapy should be determined by a consensus of the surgeon, anesthesiologist, cardiologist, and patient, who should weigh the relative risk of bleeding with that of stent thrombosis.

Class IIb B. In patients undergoing nonemergency or nonurgent noncardiac surgery who have not had previous coronary stenting, it may be reasonable to continue aspirin when the risk of potential increased cardiac events outweighs the risk of increased bleeding.

Class III B, C. Initiation or continuation of aspirin is not beneficial in patients undergoing elective noncardiac noncarotid surgery who have not had previous coronary stenting (level of evidence B) unless the risk of ischemic events outweighs the risk of surgical bleeding (level of evidence C).

The 2014 ACC/AHA guidelines recommend against routine aspirin therapy in noncardiac surgery patients who have not undergone percutaneous coronary intervention (PCI) unless risk of ischemic events is greater than the risk of surgical bleeding. These recommendations are based on evidence set forth by the POISE-2 trial. The POISE-2 trial investigated aspirin effects in noncardiac surgery. Subjects were classified based on previous exposure to aspirin either to initiation or continuation stratums. The initiation group (no previous exposure to aspirin) was randomized to aspirin or placebo starting the day of surgery and extending to 30 postoperatively. In the continuation group (subjects previously taking aspirin), subjects were randomized to either aspirin or placebo on the day of surgery and continued for 7 days postoperatively, after which they resumed their original dose of aspirin. Primary endpoints analyzed were death or nonfatal myocardial infarction within the first 30 days postoperatively. The investigators demonstrated that aspirin did not decrease either primary endpoint (HR 0.99); however, there was a statistically significant increased risk of major bleeding (HR 1.23) [33].

For patients who have undergone recent PCI, risk of in-stent thrombosis is exceedingly high and extensive recommendations have been given for this patient population. For urgent noncardiac surgery less than 6 weeks after PCI, regardless of type of stent, DAPT, consisting of aspirin and a P2Y12 inhibitor should be continued unless risk of bleeding is prohibitive [34]. For patients on DAPT who are to undergo noncardiac surgeries that require holding P2Y12 inhibitor, aspirin should be continued throughout perioperative period. A decision regarding management of antiplatelet therapy for patients who have undergone PCI should be had involving the surgeon, cardiologist, anesthesiologist, and patient.

The Clopidogrel in Unstable angina to prevent Recurrent ischemic Events (CURE) study demonstrated that the addition of clopidogrel to aspirin resulted in significantly decreased ischemic events, stroke, myocardial infarction, and death [35], resulting in wide-spread acceptance of clopidogrel as an agent of DAPT. Aspirin together with clopidogrel is now considered standard of care in prevention of in stent thrombosis in patients who have received PCI. Current guidelines suggest 12 months of DAPT (aspirin + P2Y12 receptor inhibitor) following placement of a DES in patients not at high risk for bleeding [36]. The optimal duration of DAPT is currently under investigation. A recent meta-analysis, performed on 9 randomized clinical trials involving more than 17,000 subjects demonstrated no difference in all-cause mortality, myocardial infarction, cardiac death, stent thrombosis, or cerebrovascular accidents when comparing differences in treatment duration of 12 months or more of DAPT versus therapy lasting 6 months [37,38]. Additionally, several other studies have not seen significant differences between therapy at 6 months versus 12 months or more in subjects on DAPT [39–41]. However, despite these findings, more studies are needed to delineate the appropriate length of DAPT and current guidelines still emphasize 12 months of DAPT for DES and 4 weeks for bare metal stent. Aspirin for use in primary prevention of cardiovascular disease is not as well elucidated as its use in secondary prevention and is advocated to be made on an individualized basis [13].

Significant confusion exists regarding antiplatelet agents and invasive central, neuraxial procedures. Table 3 outlines the American Society of Regional Anesthesia's (ASRA) periprocedural recommendations for cessation and resumption of antiplatelet agents for intermediate risk invasive procedures, including thoracic epidurals, lumbar epidural, intrathecal injections, and paravertebral blocks [31,34].

Anticoagulants

Overview and pharmacology

For many years, warfarin (Coumadin) has been the primary medication used in anticoagulation for many indications. Warfarin, a coumarin derivative, acts

Table 3
American Society of Regional Anesthesia recommendations for neuraxial procedure in patients taking antiplatelet therapies

Antiplatelet Agent	Recommended Interval Between Cessation of Drug and Neuraxial Block of Catheter Removal	Recommended Interval For Continuation of Drug
Aspirin	No restriction	No restriction
NSAIDS	No restriction	No restriction
Clopidogrel (Plavix)	7 d	12–24 h
Prasugrel (Effient)	7–10 d	6 h
Ticlopidine (Ticlid)	14 d	No recommendation
Abciximab (ReoPro)	2–5 d	8–12 h
Eptifibatide (Integrilin)	8–24 h	8–12 h
Tirofiban (Aggrastat)	8–24 h	8–12 h
Ticagrelor (Brilinta)	5–7 d	6 h

via inhibition of the production of vitamin K–dependent coagulation factors (II, VII, IX, X). Warfarin binds by inhibiting carboxylation and activation of vitamin K–dependent proteins [38]. Although it has been the mainstay of anticoagulation therapy, warfarin has been plagued by many problems, including variability in individual response, fluctuations in plasma levels, and decreased efficacy due to dietary effects (foods high in vitamin K), need for frequent laboratory monitoring, narrow therapeutic index, and alterations of plasma levels by many other drugs (eg, cimetidine, carbamazepine, amiodarone). These complications have led to the development of many other classes of anticoagulants that are less prone to issues that are known as non-vitamin K antagonist oral anticoagulants (NOACs).

Warfarin monitoring has traditionally been tested via the prothrombin time (PT). The PT monitors 3 vitamin K–dependent coagulation factors (II, VII, X) [38]. Due to the imprecise nature of the PT and varying laboratory differences, the International Normalized Ratio (INR) was developed to standardize reporting and is most commonly used to titrate warfarin dosages.

Nonemergent reversal of warfarin-induced bleeding can be treated with oral, intramuscular, or parenteral vitamin K. For emergent reversal of warfarin-induced bleeding, fresh frozen plasma or prothrombin concentrate (PCCs) can be used.

Indications for warfarin include most any indication for anticoagulation, including atrial fibrillation with a high CHADS2-VASC score, prevention and treatment of thromboembolic disease, prosthetic valves, procoagulant disorders (eg, lupus anticoagulant, factor V Leiden), and patients with concern for intracardiac thrombus formation due to severely depressed ventricular function.

The NOACs have several classifications based on their therapeutic mechanism. Direct thrombin inhibitors (DTIs) target thrombin (factor IIa) and inhibit coagulation by inhibiting the conversion of fibrinogen to fibrin, which strengthens clot formation. Dabigatran (Pradaxa) is the most common DTI and is indicated for atrial fibrillation not due to a heart valve issue and treatment of deep venous thrombosis and pulmonary embolism. The Randomized Evaluation of Long-Term Anticoagulant Therapy (RE-LY) trial showed that dabigatran was superior to warfarin in preventing stroke and thromboembolism without increased bleeding (3.36% with warfarin vs 3.11% with dabigatran) [42].

Monitoring of DTIs is most easily performed by activated partial thromboplastin time (aPTT) laboratory assessment. The effect of dabigatran and aPTT is curvilinear and, thus, less accurate at higher drug concentrations. The aPTT assessment of dabigatran is quantitatively limited, but can provide qualitative information in emergency situations; that is, with a normal aPTT, dabigatran-induced bleeding is unlikely to be occurring versus an elevated aPTT, which may point to increased risk of bleeding associated with elevated dabigatran levels [43]. Other laboratory tests, including thrombin time and ecarin clotting time, have been evaluated for dabigatran monitoring; however, they are not standardized nor are they widely available, making them less desirable measures [43,44].

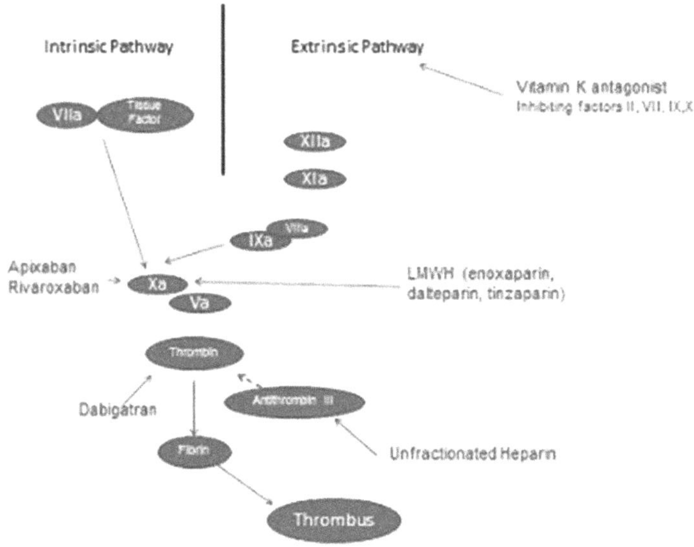

Fig. 3. Location of clotting pathway antagonism by various pharmacologic agents. LMWH, low molecular weight heparin.

Factor Xa inhibitors are another class of NOACs that directly inhibit factor Xa. Factor Xa is the first factor of the common pathway at the confluence of the intrinsic and extrinsic pathways (Fig. 3). Factor Xa leads to the ultimate production of thrombin (factor II), which leads to fibrinogen cleavage into fibrin. Currently available drugs from this class include rivaroxaban (Xarelto) and apixaban (Eliquis). The Rivaroxaban Once Daily Oral Direct factor Xa Inhibitor Compared With Vitamin K Antagonism for Prevention of Stroke and Embolism Trial in Atrial Fibrillation (ROCKET AF) demonstrated noninferiority of rivaroxaban to warfarin in stroke and thromboembolism prevention [45].

Xa inhibitors are best monitored via chromogenic anti-Xa assay, which is the standard for quantitative analysis. Unfortunately, anti-Xa assays are not widely available, thus limiting their utility. PT can be used as a qualitative screening test but depends on the reagent used. Caution should be taken not to use INR for monitoring [43].

Current guidelines and recommendations

Class I (A or B). For patients with nonvalvular atrial fibrillation with prior stroke, transient ischemic attack, or a CHADS2-VASC score of 2 or greater, oral anticoagulants are recommended. Options include warfarin (INR 2–3) (level A), dabigatran (level B), or apixaban (level B).

Class I B. For patients with atrial fibrillation who have mechanical heart valves, warfarin is recommended and the target INR (2–3 vs 2.5–3.5) should be based on type and location of the prosthesis.

Class I, C. In patients with atrial fibrillation, antithrombotic therapy should be individualized based on shared decision-making after discussion of absolute and relative risks of stroke and bleeding and the patient's values and preferences.

Class I C. For patients with nonvalvular atrial fibrillation unable to maintain therapeutic INR with warfarin, use of a direct thrombin or factor Xa inhibitor (dabigatran, rivaroxaban, or apixaban) is recommended.

Reversal of NOACs has proven to be challenging. Unlike vitamin K antagonists, no specific antidote exists and factors replaced via PCCs or plasma are inhibited by NOACs still in the circulation. In the instance of severe or life-threatening bleeding, supportive measures should be instituted with prohemostatic factors infused by prothrombin complex concentrate, antifibrinolytic therapy, or activated charcoal if ingestion occurred less than 2 hours before presentation. Dialysis may be considered in the case of bleeding associated with dabigatran, especially if renal function is depressed [43]. Specific antidotes are being developed for NOACs with idarucizumab (Praxbind) being the only one approved by the Food and Drug Administration as a reversal agent for dabigatran. This agent binds dabigatran with significantly greater affinity than thrombin, thus preventing thrombin's neutralization [44]. Andexanet alfa, currently in clinical trials, is being developed as an antidote for all factor Xa inhibitors.

Significant confusion exists surrounding anticoagulant agents, NOACs, and invasive central and neuraxial procedures. Table 4 outlines the ASRA periprocedural recommendations for cessation and resumption of anticoagulant

Table 4
American Society of Regional Anesthesia guidelines for neuraxial management in patients on anticoagulant therapies

Anticoagulant	Recommended Interval Between Cessation of Drug and Neuraxial Block or Catheter Removal	Recommended Interval for Continuation of Drug After Block
Coumadin (Warfarin)	5 d (normal INR)	24 h
Heparin (IV)	4 h (normal aPTT)	2 h
Heparin (subcutaneous)—bid and tid dosing	8–10 h	2 h
Low Molecular Weight Heparin (therapeutic dosing)	24 h	24 h
Low Molecular Weight Heparin (prophylactic dosing)	12 h	12 h
Dabigatran (Pradaxa)	5 d (6 d if impaired renal function)	24 h
Rivaroxaban (Xarelto)	3 d	24 h
Apixaban (Eliquis)	3–5 d	24 h

agents for intermediate-risk invasive procedures, including thoracic epidurals, lumbar epidural, intrathecal injections, paravertebral blocks [31,34].

References

[1] CDC. Leading causes of death. Centers for Disease Control and Prevention; 2016.
[2] Correction. Circulation 2015;131:e535.
[3] Heidenreich PA, Trogdon JG, Khavjou OA, et al. Forecasting the future of cardiovascular disease in the United States: a policy statement from the American Heart Association. Circulation 2011;123:933–44.
[4] Stone NJ, Robinson JG, Lichtenstein AH, et al. 2013 ACC/AHA guideline on the treatment of blood cholesterol to reduce atherosclerotic cardiovascular risk in adults: a report of the American College of Cardiology/American Heart Association Task Force on Practice Guidelines. J Am Coll Cardiol 2014;63:2889–934.
[5] Slater EE, MacDonald JS. Mechanism of action and biological profile of HMG CoA reductase inhibitors. A new therapeutic alternative. Drugs 1988;36(Suppl 3):72–82.
[6] Osaki Y, Nakagawa Y, Miyahara S, et al. Skeletal muscle-specific HMG-CoA reductase knockout mice exhibit rhabdomyolysis: A model for statin-induced myopathy. Biochem Biophys Res Commun 2015;466:536–40.
[7] Fleisher LA, Fleischmann KE, Auerbach AD, et al. 2014 ACC/AHA guideline on perioperative cardiovascular evaluation and management of patients undergoing noncardiac surgery: executive summary: a report of the American College of Cardiology/American Heart Association Task Force on practice guidelines. Developed in collaboration with the American College of Surgeons, American Society of Anesthesiologists, American Society of Echocardiography, American Society of Nuclear Cardiology, Heart Rhythm Society, Society for Cardiovascular Angiography and Interventions, Society of Cardiovascular Anesthesiologists, and Society of Vascular Medicine Endorsed by the Society of Hospital Medicine. J Nucl Cardiol 2015;22:162–215.
[8] Lindenauer PK, Pekow P, Wang K, et al. Lipid-lowering therapy and in-hospital mortality following major noncardiac surgery. JAMA 2004;291:2092–9.
[9] Raju MG, Pachika A, Punnam SR, et al. Statin therapy in the reduction of cardiovascular events in patients undergoing intermediate-risk noncardiac, nonvascular surgery. Clin Cardiol 2013;36:456–61.
[10] Antoniou GA, Hajibandeh S, Hajibandeh S, et al. Meta-analysis of the effects of statins on perioperative outcomes in vascular and endovascular surgery. J Vasc Surg 2015;61: 519–32.e511.
[11] Layton JB, Hansen MK, Jakobsen CJ, et al. Statin initiation and acute kidney injury following elective cardiovascular surgery: a population cohort study in Denmarkdagger. Eur J Cardiothorac Surg 2016;49:995–1000.
[12] Abramov D, Carson PE. The role of angiotensin receptor blockers in reducing the risk of cardiovascular disease. J Renin Angiotensin Aldosterone Syst 2012;13:317–27.
[13] Ferrario CM, Strawn WB. Role of the renin-angiotensin-aldosterone system and proinflammatory mediators in cardiovascular disease. Am J Cardiol 2006;98:121–8.
[14] Comfere T, Sprung J, Kumar MM, et al. Angiotensin system inhibitors in a general surgical population. Anesth Analg 2005;100:636–44.
[15] Turan A, You J, Shiba A, et al. Angiotensin converting enzyme inhibitors are not associated with respiratory complications or mortality after noncardiac surgery. Anesth Analg 2012;114:552–60.
[16] Kheterpal S, Khodaparast O, Shanks A, et al. Chronic angiotensin-converting enzyme inhibitor or angiotensin receptor blocker therapy combined with diuretic therapy is associated with increased episodes of hypotension in noncardiac surgery. J Cardiothorac Vasc Anesth 2008;22:180–6.

[17] Rosenman DJ, McDonald FS, Ebbert JO, et al. Clinical consequences of withholding versus administering renin-angiotensin-aldosterone system antagonists in the preoperative period. J Hosp Med 2008;3:319–25.
[18] Aizawa H, Imai S, Fushimi K. Factors associated with 30-day readmission of patients with heart failure from a Japanese administrative database. BMC Cardiovasc Disord 2015;15:134.
[19] Morelli A, Tritapepe L, Rocco M, et al. Terlipressin versus norepinephrine to counteract anesthesia-induced hypotension in patients treated with renin-angiotensin system inhibitors: effects on systemic and regional hemodynamics. Anesthesiology 2005;102:12–9.
[20] Wallace AW, Galindez D, Salahieh A, et al. Effect of clonidine on cardiovascular morbidity and mortality after noncardiac surgery. Anesthesiology 2004;101:284–93.
[21] Garg AX, Kurz A, Sessler DI, et al. Perioperative aspirin and clonidine and risk of acute kidney injury: a randomized clinical trial. JAMA 2014;312:2254–64.
[22] Devereaux PJ, Sessler DI, Leslie K, et al. Clonidine in patients undergoing noncardiac surgery. N Engl J Med 2014;370:1504–13.
[23] Rosendorff C, Black HR, Cannon CP, et al. Treatment of hypertension in the prevention and management of ischemic heart disease: a scientific statement from the American Heart Association Council for High Blood Pressure Research and the Councils on Clinical Cardiology and Epidemiology and Prevention. Circulation 2007;115:2761–88.
[24] Ripley TL, Saseen JJ. Beta-blockers: a review of their pharmacological and physiological diversity in hypertension. Ann Pharmacother 2014;48:723–33.
[25] Frishman WH, Saunders E. Beta-Adrenergic blockers. J Clin Hypertens (Greenwich) 2011;13:649–53.
[26] Devereaux PJ, Yang H, Yusuf S, et al. Effects of extended-release metoprolol succinate in patients undergoing non-cardiac surgery (POISE trial): a randomised controlled trial. Lancet 2008;371:1839–47.
[27] Wijeysundera DN, Duncan D, Nkonde-Price C, et al. Perioperative beta blockade in noncardiac surgery: a systematic review for the 2014 ACC/AHA guideline on perioperative cardiovascular evaluation and management of patients undergoing noncardiac surgery: a report of the American College of Cardiology/American Heart Association Task Force on practice guidelines. J Am Coll Cardiol 2014;64:2406–25.
[28] Kristensen SD, Knuuti J, Saraste A, et al. 2014 ESC/ESA Guidelines on non-cardiac surgery: cardiovascular assessment and management: The Joint Task Force on non-cardiac surgery: cardiovascular assessment and management of the European Society of Cardiology (ESC) and the European Society of Anaesthesiology (ESA). Eur J Anaesthesiol 2014;31: 517–73.
[29] Davies MJ, Thomas A. Thrombosis and acute coronary-artery lesions in sudden cardiac ischemic death. N Engl J Med 1984;310:1137–40.
[30] Hennekens CH, Dalen JE. Aspirin in the primary prevention of cardiovascular disease: current knowledge and future research needs. Trends Cardiovasc Med 2014;24:360–6.
[31] Narouze S, Benzon HT, Provenzano DA, et al. Interventional spine and pain procedures in patients on antiplatelet and anticoagulant medications: guidelines from the American Society of Regional Anesthesia and Pain Medicine, the European Society of Regional Anaesthesia and Pain Therapy, the American Academy of Pain Medicine, the International Neuromodulation Society, the North American Neuromodulation Society, and the World Institute of Pain. Reg Anesth Pain Med 2015;40:182–212.
[32] Andell P, James SK, Cannon CP, et al. Ticagrelor Versus Clopidogrel in Patients With Acute Coronary Syndromes and Chronic Obstructive Pulmonary Disease: An Analysis From the Platelet Inhibition and Patient Outcomes (PLATO) Trial. J Am Heart Assoc 2015;4:e002490.
[33] Devereaux PJ, Mrkobrada M, Sessler DI, et al. Aspirin in patients undergoing noncardiac surgery. N Engl J Med 2014;370:1494–503.
[34] Fleisher LA, Fleischmann KE, Auerbach AD, et al. 2014 ACC/AHA Guideline on Perioperative Cardiovascular Evaluation and Management of Patients Undergoing Noncardiac

Surgery: a Report of the American College of Cardiology/American Heart Association Task Force on Practice Guidelines. J Am Coll Cardiol 2014;64:e77–137.
[35] Fox KA, Mehta SR, Peters R, et al. Benefits and risks of the combination of clopidogrel and aspirin in patients undergoing surgical revascularization for non-ST-elevation acute coronary syndrome: the Clopidogrel in Unstable angina to prevent Recurrent ischemic Events (CURE) Trial. Circulation 2004;110:1202–8.
[36] Levine GN, Bates ER, Blankenship JC, et al. 2011 ACCF/AHA/SCAI Guideline for Percutaneous Coronary Intervention: executive summary: a report of the American College of Cardiology Foundation/American Heart Association Task Force on Practice Guidelines and the Society for Cardiovascular Angiography and Interventions. Catheter Cardiovasc Interv 2012;79:453–95.
[37] Pandit A, Giri S, Hakim FA, et al. Shorter (</=6 months) versus longer (>/=12 months) duration dual antiplatelet therapy after drug eluting stents: a meta-analysis of randomized clinical trials. Catheter Cardiovasc Interv 2015;85:34–40.
[38] Hirsh J, Fuster V, Ansell J, et al. American Heart Association/American College of Cardiology Foundation guide to warfarin therapy. J Am Coll Cardiol 2003;41:1633–52.
[39] Gwon HC, Hahn JY, Park KW, et al. Six-month versus 12-month dual antiplatelet therapy after implantation of drug-eluting stents: the Efficacy of Xience/Promus Versus Cypher to Reduce Late Loss After Stenting (EXCELLENT) randomized, multicenter study. Circulation 2012;125:505–13.
[40] Tada T, Natsuaki M, Morimoto T, et al. Duration of dual antiplatelet therapy and long-term clinical outcome after coronary drug-eluting stent implantation: landmark analyses from the CREDO-Kyoto PCI/CABG Registry Cohort-2. Circ Cardiovasc Interv 2012;5:381–91.
[41] Valgimigli M, Campo G, Monti M, et al. Short- versus long-term duration of dual-antiplatelet therapy after coronary stenting: a randomized multicenter trial. Circulation 2012;125:2015–26.
[42] Connolly SJ, Ezekowitz MD, Yusuf S, et al. Dabigatran versus warfarin in patients with atrial fibrillation. N Engl J Med 2009;361:1139–51.
[43] Vanden Daelen S, Peetermans M, Vanassche T, et al. Monitoring and reversal strategies for new oral anticoagulants. Expert Rev Cardiovasc Ther 2015;13:95–103.
[44] Enriquez A, Lip GY, Baranchuk A. Anticoagulation reversal in the era of the non-vitamin K oral anticoagulants. Europace 2016;18:955–64.
[45] Patel MR, Mahaffey KW, Garg J, et al. Rivaroxaban versus warfarin in nonvalvular atrial fibrillation. N Engl J Med 2011;365:883–91.

Advances in Anesthesia 34 (2016) 181–196

ADVANCES IN ANESTHESIA

Contemporary Perioperative and Anesthetic Management of Pheochromocytoma and Paraganglioma

Francis V. Salinas, MD[a,b,*]

[a]Physician Anesthesia Services, Inc, Swedish Medical Center, 1229 Madison Street, Suite 1440, Seattle, WA 98104, USA; [b]Department of Anesthesiology and Pain Medicine, University of Washington, Box 356540, 1959 Northeast Pacific Street, BB-1469, Seattle, WA 98195-6540, USA

Keywords

• Pheochromocytoma • Paraganglioma • α-blockade • Catecholamine
• Phenoxybenzamine • Prazosin • Doxazosin

Key points

- The care of patients with pheochromocytoma and paraganglioma (PPGL) presenting for surgical resection presents a challenge for the anesthesiologist.
- There is no evidence to specifically recommend the choice of preoperative pharmacologic preparation.
- Practical considerations for choice of preoperative pharmacological management include drug availability and cost.
- A detailed understanding of catecholamine biosynthesis, metabolism, and physiology provides a sound basis for understanding the cardiovascular manifestations and risks, diagnostic evaluation, preoperative preparation, and perioperative hemodynamic management of patients with PPGL presenting for surgical resection.
- Knowledge of the preoperative risk factors and perioperative events that increase the risk for hemodynamic instability provides a sound physiologic and pharmacologic basis for optimizing perioperative outcome.

Disclosure: The author has no financial relationship with a commercial company that has a direct financial interest in the subject matter or materials discussed in this article or with a company making a competing product.

*Physician Anesthesia Services, Inc, Swedish Medical Center, Seattle, WA. *E-mail address*: fvsalinasmd@gmail.com

http://dx.doi.org/10.1016/j.aan.2016.08.001

INTRODUCTION

Pheochromocytomas are catecholamine-secreting tumors that arise from the chromaffin cells located within the adrenal medulla. Paragangliomas are also catecholamine-secreting tumors arising from extra-adrenal chromaffin cells located along the sympathetic paravertebral ganglia of the pelvis, abdomen, and thorax. They are clinically relevant in perioperative medicine because they can produce and secrete large amounts of one or more catecholamines: epinephrine (E), norepinephrine (NE), and, uncommonly, dopamine. Because they produce clinically similar symptoms based on the type, amount, and secretory pattern of excess catecholamine secretion, they may be collectively referred to as pheochromocytoma and paraganglioma (PPGL).

The majority (80%–85%) of PPGL are located within the adrenal gland. PPGL are rare, with annual estimated yearly incidence of 2 to 8 cases per million [1], whereas the prevalence as a cause of secondary hypertension in the outpatient population has been estimated to be 0.1% to 0.6% [2,3]. The historically quoted "*Rule of 10s*" (10% of PPGL are extra-adrenal, 10% are malignant, 10% are bilateral, and 10% are familial) is incorrect particularly in that at least 32% of PPGL are familial [4]. In addition, the prevalence of metastatic disease varies between 10% and 17%, and in certain inherited subtypes of PPGL, the prevalence may be as high 40% or more of patients [5].

CATECHOLAMINE SYNTHESIS, METABOLISM, AND PHYSIOLOGY

A basic knowledge of the synthesis, secretion, metabolism, and physiologic actions of catecholamines is essential to understanding the clinical presentation, diagnostic evaluation, and perioperative pharmacologic management of cardiovascular manifestations of PPGL (Fig. 1) [6,7]. Catecholamines are synthesized within and subsequently secreted from chromaffin cells. The initial and rate-limiting step in catecholamine synthesis is the enzymatic hydroxylation of L-tyrosine to L-3,4-dihydroxyphenylalanine (DOPA) by tyrosine hydroxylase. Subsequently, DOPA undergoes decarboxylation by aromatic L-amino acid decarboxylase (AADC) to dopamine. Dopamine is then actively transported into

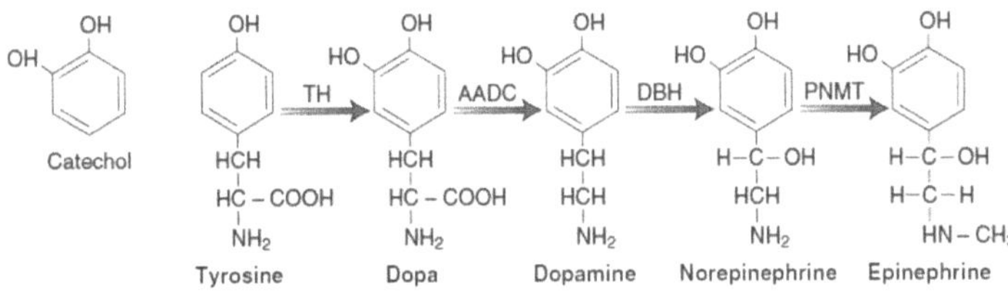

Fig. 1. Biosynthetic pathway for catecholamine metabolism. (*Modified from* Dluhy RG, Lawrence JE, Williams GH. Endocrine hypertension. In: Larsen PR, Kronenberg HM, Melmed S, et al. editors. Williams textbook of endocrinology. 10th edition. Philadelphia: Saunders; 2003. p. 555; with permission.)

neurosecretory vesicles, where it undergoes hydroxylation to NE by dopamine ß-hydroxylase. Within the adrenal medulla, NE is released back into the cytoplasm of the chromaffin cells, where it is converted to E by phenylethanolamine-*N*-methyltransferase (PNMT). E is subsequently transported back into another storage vesicle. The PNMT activity within paraganglial chromaffin cells is negligible. Therefore, catecholamine-secreting tumors that secrete predominantly E are almost always located in the adrenal medulla.

Catecholamines have a biological plasma half-life of 10 to 100 seconds, with approximately 50% loosely bound to albumin. Catecholamines are rapidly removed from the circulation by either reuptake into nerve terminals or by enzymatic methylation, conjugation, and subsequent renal excretion. Catechol-*O*-methyltransferase (COMT) converts E into metanephrine and NE into normetanephrine (Fig. 2) [6]. Metanephrine and normetanephrine are subsequently oxidized by monoamine oxidase (MAO) to vanillymandelic acid (VMA). MAO may also directly oxidize E and NE to 3,4-dihydroxymandelic acid, which is subsequently converted by COMT to VMA. MAO and COMT metabolize dopamine to homovanillic acid (HVA).

Catecholamines mediate their cardiovascular actions through binding and activation of adrenergic receptors and their specific subtypes (α_1, α_2, β_1, β_2, D_1, and D_2) [7]. NE mediates its cardiovascular effects through α_1-, α_2-, and β_1-adrenergic receptors, whereas E primarily stimulates β_1 and β_2 receptors. Postsynaptic α_1-adrenergic receptors are located on vascular smooth muscle tissue, with stimulation causing vasoconstriction of peripheral arteries and veins, increasing blood pressure. In addition, stimulation of cardiac

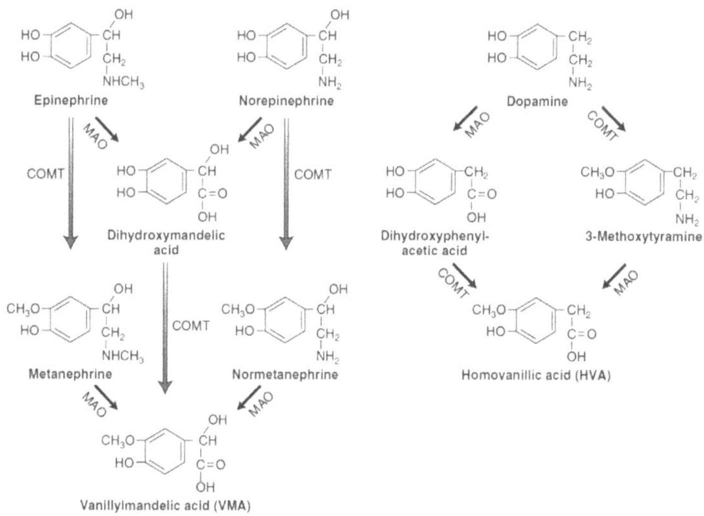

Fig. 2. Catecholamine metabolism. (*Modified from* Dluhy RG, Lawrence JE, Williams GH. Endocrine hypertension. In: Larsen PR, Kronenberg HM, Melmed S, et al. editors. Williams textbook of endocrinology. 10th edition. Philadelphia: Saunders; 2003. p. 556; with permission.)

myocyte α_1-adrenergic receptors has positive inotropic effects. α_2-Adrenergic receptors are located on the presynaptic sympathetic nerve terminals, and when activated, provide a negative feedback loop for NE release, resulting in inhibition of central sympathetic outflow and decreased blood pressure.

β_1-Adrenergic receptor activation produces increased inotropic and chronotropic effects on the heart, increased renin secretion (increasing blood pressure by converting angiotensin to angiotensin-1) in the kidney, and increased lipolysis. β_2-Adrenergic receptor activation produces vascular smooth muscle relaxation and results in bronchodilation, vasodilation in skeletal muscle arteries, increased release of NE from sympathetic nerve terminals, as well as increased glycogenolysis. D_1-adrenergic receptors are located on cerebral, renal, and mesenteric arteries, and stimulation causes vasodilation in these vascular beds.

CLINICAL PRESENTATION

The most common symptom of PPGL is hypertension, found in approximately 95% of patients. PPGL may also present with the classic symptom triad of headache, palpitations, and diaphoresis [8]. The clinical presentation of hypertension varies widely and displays either a sustained or a paroxysmal pattern depending on multiple factors, including the amount and timing of catecholamine production and secretion. Sustained hypertension is typical of NE-secreting tumors and, in contrast, orthostatic hypotension (lightheadedness, presyncope, or syncope) may characterize the clinical presentation of predominantly E-secreting or dopamine-secreting tumors [9]. Other nonspecific symptoms include nausea, anorexia, anxiety, lethargy, tremor, and hyperglycemia. Abdominal pain or chest pain may also be present secondary to arterial vasoconstriction. Patients may also present with pheochromocytoma crisis, manifesting most commonly with acute cardiac symptoms such as cardiomyopathy (Takotsubo), myocardial infarction, or cardiogenic shock [10]. In contrast, approximately 50% of PPGL are initially discovered incidentally on abdominal imaging for an unrelated indication.

The most common reason patients with PPGL are encountered by an anesthesiologist is for surgical excision of the tumor. Although the diagnosis should be well established before the patient presents for adrenalectomy, it is important for the anesthesiologist to have a detailed understanding of the diagnostic workup, goals, and rationale of preoperative preparation (including choice of preoperative α- and/or β-blockade), indications and implications for laparoscopic versus open adrenalectomy, and risk factors for perioperative hemodynamic instability (HDI), which can include severe hypertension and/or postresection hypotension.

DIAGNOSTIC WORKUP FOR PHEOCHROMOCYTOMA AND PARAGANGLIOMA

Biochemical testing

The traditional biochemical diagnosis of pheochromocytoma used to rely on random plasma and 24-hour urine collections for analysis of urinary total and fractionated (E, NE, and dopamine) catecholamines [11,12]. However, the short half-life of plasma catecholamines makes it difficult to differentiate pathologic excess production-secretion from a transient stress response such as venipuncture [13]. In contrast, catecholamine metabolism is constant, with the sulfated metabolites (metanephrine and normetanephrine) having long half-lives, and eventually excretion in the urine. Thus, more contemporary diagnostic techniques should include measurements of plasma-free metanephrine and normetanephrine as well as 24-hour urine collection for fractionated metanephrine and metanephrine and normetanephrine [11,12,14]. Although plasma-free fractionated metanephrines have a higher sensitivity (96%–100% vs 86%–97%) and specificity (89%–96% vs 86%–95%) compared with urinary fractionated metanephrines, there is no consensus on which test is superior [8,14]. Dopamine-secreting tumors can be measured by measuring plasma and urinary dopamine and HVA levels.

Imaging

Either before, or more commonly after, confirmatory biochemical diagnosis, imaging plays a critical role in characterizing tumor location (as well as differentiating unilateral vs bilateral disease) and size. Computed tomography (CT) and MRI have comparable sensitivity, but MRI is superior in identifying paragangliomas and has a higher specificity than CT [6,14]. Additional functional imaging (scintigraphy) using radiotracers ($MIBG^{123}$ [meta-iodobenzylguanidine], which concentrates in adrenergic tissue after ingestion) is particularly useful when CT/MRI results are equivocal and to detect possible lesions (metastatic disease) distant from the primary adrenal location, or for localizing paragangliomas.

PREOPERATIVE MANAGEMENT

From the perspective of an anesthesiologist, the principal goal in the preoperative management of patients with PPGL is to minimize the severity, duration, and frequency of HDI that is likely to be encountered during the perioperative management of surgical resection (either open or laparoscopic approach). The preoperative preparation of patients will typically require a multidisciplinary approach between the primary surgical team, the referring endocrinologist, cardiology (if preoperative cardiac evaluation is required), and the anesthesiologist. Ideally, the anesthesiologist will have detailed knowledge of the patient's planned surgical date and approach, adequacy of preoperative preparation, and an understanding of the risk factors for HDI during the perioperative period. It has been the practice of the author to have the surgeon and/or endocrinologist refer the patient to the anesthesia department for formal preoperative consultation and, in most cases, to assume management and titration of preoperative pharmacologic (α-adrenergic blockade) management in the 2 to 3 weeks before surgery.

The principal goals in the preoperative management include the following [8,14]:

1. Blood pressure control
2. Repletion of chronic intravascular volume depletion

3. Control of heart rate and associated tachyarrhythmia
4. Assessment and optimization of associated metabolic disturbances
5. Assessment and optimization of myocardial function

PREOPERATIVE BLOOD PRESSURE CONTROL

Although there is a lack of rigorous evidence (in the form of randomized controlled trials) and the evidence base (in the form of multiple retrospective reviews, case series, and case controlled series) has recently been questioned [15], institution of preoperative α-blockade is currently recommended for all patients before adrenalectomy [8,14]. Current consensus guidelines recommend at least 7 to 14 days to allow adequate time to normalize blood pressure and heart rate [14]. Chronic vasoconstriction from catecholamine excess results in an intravascular volume-depleted state. Although lacking rigorous data, a rational approach to correct preoperative hypovolemia is to have the patient institute a high sodium diet and encourage liberal fluid intake, but only after adequate blood pressure control has been obtained. Caution regarding instituting aggressive volume repletion is warranted in patients with compromised ventricular systolic or diastolic function. There is lack of rigorous evidence to determine the optimal target blood pressure and heart rate. Based on several retrospective studies, the current recommendations aim for target blood pressure of less than 130/85 mm Hg while seated and greater than 90 mm Hg systolic [14]. The current recommendations recommend a target heart rate of 60 to 70 beats per minute while seated and 70 to 80 beats per minute while standing. Previous recommendations that orthostatic hypotension (with at least a 15% decrease in blood pressure, but not <80 mm Hg systolic) was an indicator of optimal blockade should be questioned [16]. Orthostatic hypotension should not be considered a goal of treatment, but rather a side effect of the institution and achievement of adequate α-adrenergic blockade in the setting of catecholamine-induced chronic vasoconstriction.

α-ADRENERGIC BLOCKADE

Although preoperative α-adrenergic blockade is recommended for all patients undergoing adrenalectomy in patients with PPGL, there is still a lack of consensus on the optimal choice of α-adrenergic blocking drug. Historically, phenoxybenzamine had been the most widely used α-blocking agent used for the preoperative preparation of patients with PPGL. Phenoxybenzamine is a noncompetitive and nonselective α-adrenergic antagonist that covalently binds to both α_1 and α_2 receptors. The typical starting dose is 10 mg/d and is increased until adequate blood pressure control is obtained. Generally, a total dose of 1 mg/kg per day (in 2–3 divided doses) is sufficient to achieve optimal α-blockade [8]. The theoretical advantage of the noncompetitive action of phenoxybenzamine is that even when excessive amounts of catecholamines are released (as commonly occurs during surgical manipulation), phenoxybenzamine will not be displaced, thus minimizing hypertensive responses. The noncompetitive nature results in a prolonged duration of action as de novo synthesis of α-adrenergic receptors is required. This property may potentially lead to prolonged postoperative refractory (catecholamine-resistant) hypotension. An additional disadvantage of the nonspecific blockade of phenoxybenzamine is the high incidence of reflex tachycardia due to blockade (inhibition) of presynaptic α_2 receptors, which inhibits the normal negative feedback loop that regulates NE release. The tachycardia induced by α-blockade, however, indicates that adequate α-blockade has been achieved. Therefore, a β-adrenergic antagonist is typically added to phenoxybenzamine therapy to decrease the chronotropic response to uninhibited NE release. Practical disadvantages for phenoxybenzamine use include nasal congestion, marked fatigue, centrally mediated sedation, and retrograde ejaculation in men. Lastly, the increasing lack of availability and its marked cost (when not covered by health insurance) are additional practical real world disadvantages of phenoxybenzamine.

The use of selective, competitive α_1-adrenergic antagonists (doxazosin and prazosin) offers several potential advantages when compared with phenoxybenzamine. They do not elicit α_2-mediated reflex tachycardia and have a relatively short duration of action as a consequence of their competitive inhibition. Doxazosin is the most commonly used agent and can be started at 1 mg/d and increased until optimal dosing (typically between 1 and 16 mg/d) is reached. Its relatively long half-life of 16 to 30 hours allows for convenient once-daily dosing. Prazosin has a much shorter half-life (3–5 hours) and typically requires 2 to 3 times daily dosing (typically 2 to 6 mg three times a day), which may allow for more rapid resolution of α-blockade after tumor devascularization. The theoretical disadvantage of competitive inhibition may be displacement by excessive catecholamine levels, resulting in less effective control (as compared with phenoxybenzamine) of hypertensive surges that may occur during surgical manipulation. There have been 8 nonrandomized studies examining the efficacy of phenoxybenzamine compared with selective α_1-competative blockers (doxazosin, terazosin, or prazosin) [17–24]. Four studies were retrospective reviews of an institutional change from phenoxybenzamine to selective α_1-competative blockers; 2 were nonrandomized in nature (α-blockade based on the discretion of either the surgical team or endocrinologist), one compared 2 different institutional protocols (phenoxybenzamine at the Mayo Clinic vs selective α_1-competative blockers at the Cleveland Clinic) [20], and, in one study, the basis for the choice of α-blockade was unclear [23]. Overall, the results of these nonrandomized controlled trials did not demonstrate a clinically relevant difference in either the frequency of severe elevations in blood pressure or the frequency of prolonged postoperative hypotension between the 2 classes of agents. The efficacy of phenoxybenzamine versus doxazosin is currently being investigated in a multicenter randomized controlled trial (PRESCRIPT) [25]. In the absence of clinically significant efficacy, secondary considerations of convenience, side-effect profile, and availability are important and practical considerations in the choice of preoperative α-blocking agent [26,27]. Perhaps more importantly in the current health care economic environment, cost may also play a role in the choice of agent. A 30-day supply of doxazosin (1–8 mg) ranges in cost from $10 to $30. In contrast, a 30-day supply of phenoxybenzamine (10 mg three times a day) costs on average $22,000 [28].

β-ADRENERGIC BLOCKADE

The principal indication for preoperative β-adrenergic antagonist therapy is to prevent or control catecholamine-induced cardiac tachyarrhythmia, which will be more evident in patients with predominantly E-secreting tumors. In addition, β-antagonist therapy is also indicated to control reflex tachycardia associated with phenoxybenzamine blockade. β-Blocker therapy should never be used as the initial antihypertensive (eg, in the absence of established α-blockade) in patients with suspected or diagnosed PPGL. β-Blocker therapy (in the absence of α_1-blockade) may potentially result in unopposed α_1-mediated vasoconstriction due to loss of β_2-mediated vasodilation and the potential for hypertensive crisis, as well as compromising myocardial function due to the negative inotropic effects of β-antagonism [29]. Because the primary indication for β-antagonist therapy is control of tachyarrhythmia, cardioselective β_1-antagonists (atenolol or metoprolol) should be used, because nonselective β-antagonist therapy may potentially antagonize β_2-mediated vasodilation. Labetalol should also be used with caution as a first-line antihypertensive in patients with PPGL. Although labetalol has both α_1-antagonist and β-antagonist activity, the fixed ratio of α_1/β-antagonist activity (1:7) when given orally may potentially result in paradoxic episodes of hypertension, or even hypertensive crisis [30].

NONADRENERGIC ANTIHYPERTENSIVE AGENTS

Calcium-channel blockers inhibit catecholamine-induced calcium influx, causing vascular smooth muscle relaxation of both peripheral and coronary arteries. They may also be used in conjunction with α- and β-antagonist therapy or, less commonly, as the primary agent for blood pressure control in patients with PPGL [31,32]. They are not recommended as monotherapy unless patients have only very mild hypertension or develop severe orthostatic hypotension with α-blockade [14]. Sustained release nicardipine (30 mg twice a day) is a commonly used preparation. Catecholamine-synthesis inhibitors may also be added in patients with PPGL with catecholamine levels that are unresponsive to α-adrenergic and calcium channel blockade [33]. α-Methyl-L-tyrosine (metyrosine) inhibits tyrosine hydroxylase, the initial and rate-limiting enzyme in catecholamine synthesis (see Fig. 1), typically reducing catecholamine stores after 3 days of therapy [8,33]. Because there is incomplete depletion of catecholamine stores, it is not effective as monotherapy and must be used in conjunction with α-adrenergic blockade [34]. Although a recently published retrospective case series demonstrated that metyrosine added to phenoxybenzamine provided better perioperative hemodynamic stability compared with phenoxybenzamine alone [33], its routine use is not recommended because of the high incidence of disabling side effects (severe sedation, depression, galactorrhea, and extrapyramidal symptoms) [8] and cost (250 mg twice a day costs approximately $22,000) [28]. Thus, it is typically reserved for patients with PPGL with widespread metastatic disease [8,14,35].

ASSESSMENT AND OPTIMIZATION OF MYOCARDIAL FUNCTION AND METABOLIC ABNORMALITIES

Preoperative cardiac evaluation should include risk assessment for ischemic heart disease secondary to either excess catecholamine levels or preexisting coronary artery disease. At a minimum, a 12-lead electrocardiogram should be reviewed for evidence of ventricular hypertrophy, tachyarrhythmia, or ongoing myocardial ischemia. Even in the absence of cardiac symptoms, all patients should have an echocardiogram to assess for ventricular systolic and diastolic function. In addition, an echocardiogram should assess for the potential presence of various forms of cardiomyopathy associated with PPGL, such as concentric hypertrophy, or less commonly, Takotsubo cardiomyopathy [36,37]. Hyperglycemia due to catecholamine excess is a common metabolic abnormality associated with PPGL [6,8]. The cause is multifactorial, occurring because of increased gluconeogenesis, glycogenolysis, and lipolysis secondary to stimulation of β-adrenergic receptors, decreased insulin release by stimulation of pancreatic α-adrenergic receptors, as well as increased glucagon release coupled with peripheral insulin resistance.

INTRAOPERATIVE MANAGEMENT

There are no data to support any specific anesthetic approach nor hemodynamic management techniques to treat perioperative hemodynamic responses (hypertension and tachycardia secondary to anesthetic management and surgical manipulation, and/or hypotension after tumor devascularization). Thus, the recommendations provided focus on identifying the risk factors for perioperative HDI as well as key aspects during anesthesia and the surgical procedure that may provoke significant hemodynamic responses.

RISK FACTORS FOR HEMODYNAMIC INSTABILITY

HDI during the course of surgical resection of PPGL remains a common occurrence even when patients have been adequately prepared (institution of α-blockade for at least 7 days before surgery and adequate intravascular volume repletion) [38]. Severe and prolonged elevations in blood pressure and/or heart rate, associated with paroxysmal severe elevations in the secretion of catecholamines, are typically associated with surgical manipulation of the tumor. Just as importantly, rapid and profound decreases in blood pressure may be seen, often occurring shortly after tumor devascularization (adrenal vein ligation) due to the abrupt decrease in circulating levels of catecholamines.

Numerous studies have attempted to identify risk factors [21,39–46] for HDI, and the most important include larger (typically defined as >6.0 cm) tumor size, significantly elevated catecholamine production, and inadequate preoperative control of blood pressure (failing to achieve <130/85 mm Hg or mean arterial pressure [MAP] < 100 mm Hg consistent with published guidelines for target goals [14]) (Box 1). Additional risk factors include symptomatically elevated blood pressure, lower doses of preoperative α-blockade, and, in one study, open instead of laparoscopic approach [21,39–46]. The common theme identified here is a high level of circulating catecholamines (or metabolites). Higher catecholamine levels at the time of diagnosis would likely present with symptoms before institution of α-blockade, and it would seem logical to assume that it would require increased doses of preoperative α-blocker (regardless of selective vs nonselective agent) to achieve normalization of blood pressure. Larger tumor size and an open approach (typically required with larger tumors) may also reflect an increased overall catecholamine burden before resection. Not surprisingly, the same risk factors that predicted elevated blood pressure during surgical resection also predicted a longer duration of postresection hypotension [46]. One of the proposed mechanisms may be that chronically marked elevations in catecholamines cause a compensatory downregulation of adrenergic receptors, resulting in a relative catecholamine resistance, and thus, exacerbating the consequences of the acute decreases in catecholamines after tumor devascularization [47].

KEY ASPECTS DURING THE SURGICAL RESECTION OF PHEOCHROMOCYTOMA AND PARAGANGLIOMA

There are no specific anesthetic techniques associated with either improved hemodynamic stability or outcome for surgical resection of PPGL. However, there are several key aspects that warrant discussion. Invasive arterial monitoring should be obtained before induction of anesthesia. Not only does direct arterial pressure monitoring provide continuous assessment of blood pressure but also analysis of systolic pressure variation may also assist with guiding fluid therapy (responsiveness) after tumor devascularization [48]. Reliable

Box 1: Risk factors for perioperative hemodynamic instability during adrenalectomy for pheochromocytoma and paraganglioma

- Larger tumor size (6.0 cm)
- Increased (>6–10 times upper limit of normal) catecholamine levels
- Increased (>6–10 times upper limit of normal) metanephrine/normetanephrine levels
- MAP > 100 mm Hg (130/85 mm Hg) before surgery
- Symptomatic[a] high preoperative blood pressure before surgery
- Lower doses of α-adrenergic blockade
- Lack of intraoperative magnesium sulfate use
- Open (vs laparoscopic) approach

[a] Permanent or paroxysmal symptoms of headache, sweating, palpitations, flushing requiring urgent medical treatment.

central venous access is recommended, if only for vasoactive infusion delivery. Transesophageal echocardiography is not mandatory, but may prove especially useful in cases of postresection catecholamine-resistant hypotension. There are no prospective randomized studies comparing laparoscopic with open adrenalectomy for PPGL. Current guidelines recommend laparoscopic resection for most patients [14]. Laparoscopic approaches are typically associated with decreased postoperative pain, decreased hospital length of stay, and less surgical morbidity compared with open approaches. However, current guidelines recommend open resection for large or locally invasive PPGL to ensure complete tumor resection, prevent tumor rupture, and avoid local recurrence [14]. Beyond these general guidelines, there are several key aspects that warrant discussion:

- Avoid medication-induced catecholamine release
- Minimize catecholamine release induced by anesthetic or surgical maneuvers
- Anticipate and minimize hemodynamic responses to paroxysmal increases in catecholamine release that may occur during tumor manipulation
- Anticipate and minimize expected hypotension after tumor devascularization
- Anticipate and plan for possible postoperative cardiovascular and metabolic complications

Avoid medication-induced catecholamine release

Numerous commonly used drugs may potentially increase catecholamine levels via multiple mechanisms. They may increase presynaptic catecholamine release, inhibit catecholamine reuptake, or cause histamine release. Medications to consider avoiding include desflurane, ephedrine, ketamine, morphine, meperidine, atracurium, pancuronium, succinylcholine, droperidol, metoclopramide, and cocaine. From a practical standpoint, it would be best to avoid inadvertent administration of E, such as with an epidural test dose, or more commonly in local anesthetic solutions, routinely used for skin infiltration before placement of laparoscopic trocars.

Minimize catecholamine release induced by anesthetic or surgical maneuvers

Although tumor manipulation induces by far the most significant potential for catecholamine release and subsequent hemodynamic responses, catecholamine release may also be provoked by direct laryngoscopy and endotracheal intubation. The creation of pneumoperitoneum predictably results in increased catecholamine release and should be taken into account by both the surgical and the anesthetic teams [49]. Careful communication between the surgical and anesthetic team during these key phases is essential. Analogous to asking the surgeon to remove a cross-clamp when there are significant hemodynamic changes seen with aortic cross-clamping, the anesthesiologist can request the surgeon to temporarily stop abdominal insufflation or tumor manipulation until the appropriate vasoactive medications can be initiated and titrated to desired effect.

Anticipate and minimize hemodynamic responses to paroxysmal increases in catecholamine release that may occur during tumor manipulation

Catecholamine surges during tumor manipulation can result in profound hypertension, tachyarrhythmia (with E-secreting tumors), or bradycardia (with NE-secreting tumors). Although early surgical ligation of the adrenal vein was traditionally recommended to attenuate catecholamine surges, this approach is associated with a higher risk of damaging surrounding structures, particularly for larger tumors. Retrospective case reviews [50,51] and a recent randomized controlled trial [52] found no difference in plasma catecholamine levels or episodes of HDI between the early or late adrenal vein ligation groups. Significant elevations in blood pressure are typically managed with a vasodilator, whereas tachyarrhythmia is controlled with a β-adrenergic antagonist. There is little evidence on which to base drug selection to control HDI. The choices should be made based on drug availability, pharmacodynamic and pharmacokinetic profiles, and familiarity with the chosen vasoactive agents. Commonly used agents to control hypertension include directing α_1-anatagonists such as phentolamine or urapidil, nitric oxide vasodilators such as sodium nitroprusside and nitroglycerin, calcium channel blockers such nicardipine or clevidipine, dopamine-1 receptor agonists (fenoldopam), and esmolol [53,54]. Older case reports, along with recent reviews, also highlight the potential for intravenous magnesium sulfate to control hemodynamic response to surgical resection [55,56].

Anticipate and minimize expected hypotension after tumor devascularization

Episodes of hypotension before tumor devascularization may result from anesthetic agents, decreased intravascular volume, and more commonly, from the treatment of a hypertensive episode outlasting a transient catecholamine surge. These transient episodes can be minimized with careful titration of vasodilators, and a combination of fluid boluses and administration of the direct-acting α_1-agonist, phenylephrine. However, hypotension seen after tumor devascularization is relatively common and may be both profound and resistant to traditional catecholamine therapy with NE and E. The underlying mechanism is multifactorial and likely includes a combination of residual α_1-adrenergic blockade (especially with preoperative use of phenoxybenzamine), abrupt catecholamine deficiency, inadequate intravascular volume (relative to abrupt venous pooling from catecholamine deficiency or absolute from surgical losses), or even catecholamine receptor downregulation [47], especially in patients with high preoperative catecholamine levels. The initial treatment should include discontinuation of vasodilator therapy, optimization of intravascular fluid volume (guided by pulse pressure variation and/or transesophageal echocardiography), and aggressive titration with NE and/or phenylephrine. If hypotension is refractory to the previous measures, vasopressin should be considered. Vasopressin causes systemic vasoconstriction by acting on systemic arterial V1 receptors [56]. Because vasopressin does not rely on the availability of adrenergic receptors for its vasopressor effect, it may be particularly suited for treatment of catecholamine-resistant hypotension during pheochromocytoma resection [57,58]. It also increases circulatory volume by acting on V2 in the distal convoluted tubule and collecting ducts of the kidney, thereby increasing water resorption [56]. The effective use of vasopressin has been shown to reverse severe hypotension successfully in patients with vasodilatory shock associated with sepsis, anaphylaxis, postcardiac bypass vasoplegia, and angiotensin receptor blockade [59].

Anticipate and plan for possible postoperative cardiovascular and metabolic complications

Most patients should continue to have invasive arterial pressure monitoring in an intensive care setting for at least 12 to 24 hours after surgery. However, it may be reasonable after a 6- to 12-hour interval of postoperative hemodynamic stability to monitor low-risk patients (uncomplicated laparoscopic surgery and absence of vasopressor use before discharge from the postanesthesia care unit) in a nonintensive care setting [43]. Postoperative hypoglycemia may also occur as a result of acute catecholamine deficiency and rebound hyperinsulinemia. The classic hyperadrenergic symptoms associated with hypoglycemia may also be masked by residual postoperative β-adrenergic blockade. Typically, this is a transient phenomenon, and close glucose monitoring (every 4–6 hours) is only required first the 24 hours after surgery. However, there are case reports of prolonged or recurrent hypoglycemia [60,61]. A recently published retrospective review of 215 patients demonstrated that the incidence (4.2%) is relatively uncommon, but may be higher in patients with E-secreting tumors [62].

SUMMARY

The care of patients with PPGL presenting for surgical resection presents a challenge for the anesthesiologist. There is no evidence to specifically recommend the choice of preoperative pharmacologic preparation. Practical considerations include drug availability and cost. A detailed understanding of catecholamine biosynthesis, metabolism, and physiology provides a sound basis for understanding the cardiovascular manifestations and risks, diagnostic evaluation, preoperative preparation, and perioperative hemodynamic management of patients with PPGL presenting for surgical resection. Knowledge of the preoperative risk factors and perioperative events that increase the risk for HDI provides a sound physiologic and pharmacologic basis for optimizing perioperative outcome.

References

[1] Stenström G, Svärdsudd K. Pheochromocytoma in Sweden 1958-1981. An analysis of the National Cancer Registry Data. Acta Med Scand 1986;220:225–32.
[2] Sinclair AM, Isles CG, Brown I, et al. Secondary hypertension in a blood pressure clinic. Arch Intern Med 1987;147:1289–93.

[3] Omura M, Saito J, Yamaguchi K, et al. Prospective study on the prevalence of secondary hypertension among hypertensive patients visiting a general outpatient clinic in Japan. Hypertens Res 2004;27:193–202.
[4] Jimenez-Roquelpo AP, Dahia PL, Robeldo M. An update on the genetics of paraganglioma, pheochromocytoma, and associated hereditary syndromes. Horm Metab Res 2012;44: 328–33.
[5] Proye C, Vix M, Goropoulos A, et al. High incidence of malignant pheochromocytoma in a surgical unit. 26 cases out of 100 patients operated from 1971 to 1991. J Endocrinol Invest 1992;15:651–63.
[6] Young WF. Endocrine hypertension. In: Melmed S, Polonsky KS, Larsen PR, et al, editors. Williams text of endocrinology. 13th edition. Philadelphia: Elsevier; 2016. p. 556–88.
[7] Eisenhofer G, Kopin IJ, Goldstein DS. Catecholamine metabolism: a contemporary view with implications for physiology and medicine. Pharmacol Rev 2004;56:331–49.
[8] Pacak K. Approach to the patient. Preoperative management of the pheochromocytoma patient. J Clin Endocrinol Metab 2007;91:4069–79.
[9] Zuber SM, Kantorovich V, Pacak K. Hypertension in pheochromocytoma: characteristics and treatment. Endocrinol Metab Clin North Am 2011;40:295–311.
[10] Whitelaw BC, Prague JK, Mustafa OG, et al. Phaeochromocytoma crisis. Clin Endocrinol (Oxf) 2014;80:13–22.
[11] van Berkel A, Lenders JW, Timmers HJ. Diagnosis of endocrine disease: biochemical diagnosis of phaeochromocytoma and paraganglioma. Eur J Endocrinol 2014;170:R109–19.
[12] Eisenhofer G, Peitzsch M. Laboratory evaluation of pheochromocytoma and paraganglioma. Clin Chem 2014;60:1486–99.
[13] Amar L, Eisenhofer G. Diagnosing pheochromocytoma-paraganglioma in a patient presenting with critical illness: biochemistry versus imaging. Clin Endocrinol 2015;83:298–302.
[14] Lenders JW, Duh QY, Eisenhofer G, et al. Pheochromocytoma and paraganglioma: an Endocrine Society clinical practice guideline. J Clin Endocrinol Metab 2014;99:1915–42.
[15] Lentschener C, Gaujoux S, Tesniere A, et al. Point of controversy: perioperative care of patients undergoing pheochromocytoma removal—time for a reappraisal? Eur J Endocrinol 2011;165:365–73.
[16] Witteles RM, Kaplan EL, Roizen MF. Safe and cost-effective preoperative preparation of patients with pheochromocytoma. Anesth Analg 2000;91:302–4.
[17] Prys-Roberts C, Farndon JR. Efficacy and safety of doxazosin for perioperative management of patients with pheochromocytoma. World J Surg 2002;26:1037–42.
[18] Kocak S, Aydintug S, Canakci N. Alpha blockade in preoperative preparation of patients with pheochromocytomas. Int Surg 2002;87:191–4.
[19] Zhu Y, He HC, Su TW, et al. Selective α_1-adrenoreceptor antagonist (controlled release tablets) in preoperative management of pheochromocytoma. Endocrine 2010;38:254–9.
[20] Weingarten TN, Cata JP, O'Hara JF, et al. Comparison of two preoperative medical management strategies for laparoscopic resection of pheochromocytoma. Urology 2010;76: 508.e6-11.
[21] Bruynzeel H, Feelders RA, Groenland TH, et al. Risk factors for hemodynamic instability during surgery for pheochromocytoma. J Clin Endocrinol Metab 2010;95:678–85.
[22] Agrawal R, Mishra SK, Bhatia E, et al. Prospective study to compare perioperative hemodynamic alterations following preparation for pheochromocytoma surgery by phenoxybenzamine or prazosin. World J Surg 2014;38:716–23.
[23] Li J, Yang CH. Improvement of preoperative management in patients with adrenal pheochromocytoma. Int J Clin Exp Med 2014;7:5541–6.
[24] Randle RW, Balentine CJ, Pitt SC, et al. Selective versus nonselective α-blockade prior to laparoscopic adrenalectomy for pheochromocytoma. Ann Surg Oncol 2016; http://dx.doi.org/10.1245/s10434-016-5514-7.
[25] Phenoxybenzamine versus doxazosin in PCC patients (PRESCRIPT). Available at: http://clinicaltrials.gov/show/NCT01379898. Accessed August 27, 2016.

[26] James M. The impact of changes in drug availability for hemodynamic management in pheochromocytoma: prêt-à-porter or tailor-made? Can J Anaesth 2015;62:1244–7.
[27] Ramichandran R, Reward V. Preoperative optimization in pheochromocytoma: phenoxybenzamine may be redundant but not alpha blockade. Can J Anaesth 2015;63:629.
[28] GoodRx, Inc. Available at: http://www.goodrx.com. Accessed August 27, 2016.
[29] Sibal L, Jovanovic A, Agarwal C, et al. Phaeochromocytomas presenting as acute crises after beta blockade therapy. Clin Endocrinol (Oxf) 2006;65:186–90.
[30] MacCarthy EP, Bloomfield SS. Labetalol: a review of its pharmacology, pharmacokinetics, clinical uses and adverse effects. Pharmacotherapy 1983;3:193–219.
[31] Brunaud L, Boutmai M, Nguyen PL, et al. Both preoperative alpha and calcium channel blockade impact intraoperative hemodynamic stability similarly in the management of pheochromocytoma. Surgery 2014;156:1410–8.
[32] Lebuffe G, Dosseh ED, Tek G, et al. The effect of calcium channel blockers on outcome following the surgical treatment of phaeochromocytomas and paragangliomas. Anaesthesia 2005;60:439–44.
[33] Wachtel H, Kennedy EH, Zaher S, et al. Preoperative metyrosine improves cardiovascular outcome for patients undergoing surgery for pheochromocytoma and paraganglioma. Ann Surg Oncol 2015;22:S646–54.
[34] Thanapaalasingham K, Pollmann AS, Schelew B. Failure of metyrosine therapy for preoperative management of pheochromocytoma: a case report. Can J Anaesth 2015;62:1303–7.
[35] Kopf D, Goretzki PE, Lehnert H. Clinical management of malignant adrenal tumors. J Cancer Res Clin Oncol 2001;127:143–55.
[36] Prejbizs A, Lenders JW, Eisenhofer G, et al. Cardiovascular manifestations of phaeochromocytoma. J Hypertens 2011;29:2049–60.
[37] Subramayan S, Kreisberg RA. Pheochromocytoma: a cause of ST-segment elevation myocardial infarction, transient left ventricular dysfunction, and Takotsubo cardiomyopathy. Endocr Pract 2012;18:e77–80.
[38] Eisenhofer G, Bornstein SR. Surgery: risk of hemodynamic instability in pheochromocytoma. Nat Rev Endocrinol 2010;6:301–2.
[39] Kinney MA, Warner ME, vanHeerden JA, et al. Perianesthetic risks and outcomes of pheochromocytoma and paraganglioma resection. Anesth Analg 2000;91:1118–23.
[40] Chang RYK, Lang BHH, Wong KP, et al. High preoperative urinary norepinephrine is an independent determinant of the perioperative hemodynamic instability in unilateral pheochromocytoma/paraganglioma removal. World J Surg 2014;38:2317–23.
[41] Kiernan CM, Du L, Chen X, et al. Predictors of hemodynamic instability during surgery for pheochromocytoma. Ann Surg Oncol 2014;21:3865–71.
[42] Livingstone M, Duttchen K, Thompson J, et al. Hemodynamic stability during pheochromocytoma resection: lessons learned over the last two decades. Ann Surg Oncol 2015;22:4175–80.
[43] Benay CE, Tahiri M, Lee L, et al. Selective strategy for intensive monitoring after pheochromocytoma resection. Surgery 2016;159:275–83.
[44] Brunaud L, Nguyen-Thi PL, Mirallie E, et al. Predictive factors for postoperative morbidity after laparoscopic adrenalectomy for pheochromocytoma: a multicenter retrospective analysis 225 patients. Surg Endosc 2016;30:1051–9.
[45] Gaujoux S, Bonnet S, Lentschener C, et al. Preoperative risk factors of hemodynamic instability during laparoscopic adrenalectomy for pheochromocytoma. Surg Endosc 2016;30:2984–93.
[46] Namekawa T, Utsumi T, Kawamura K, et al. Clinical predictors of prolonged postresection hypotension after laparoscopic adrenalectomy for pheochromocytoma. Surgery 2016;159:763–70.
[47] Cryer PE. Physiology and pathophysiology of the human sympathoadrenal neuroendocrine system. N Engl J Med 1980;303:436–44.

[48] Mallot J, Pironkov A, Destandau MS, et al. Systolic pressure variation (Deltadown) can guide fluid therapy during pheochromocytoma surgery. Can J Anaesth 2003;50: 998–1003.
[49] Joris JL, Hamoir EE, Hartsein GM, et al. Hemodynamic changes and catecholamine release during laparoscopic adrenalectomy for pheochromocytoma. Anesth Analg 1998;88: 16–21.
[50] Vassiliou MC, Laycock WS. Laparoscopic adrenalectomy for pheochromocytoma: take the vein last? Surg Endosc 2009;23:965–8.
[51] Zografos GN, Farfaras AK, Kassi E, et al. Laparoscopic resection of pheochromocytomas with delayed vein ligation. Surg Laparosc Endosc Percutan Tech 2011;21:116–9.
[52] Wu G, Zhang B, Yu C, et al. Effect of early adrenal vein ligation on blood pressure and catecholeamine fluctuation during laparoscopic adrenalectomy for pheochromocytoma. Urology 2013;82:606–11.
[53] Padilla Ramos A, Varon J. Current and newer agents for hypertensive emergencies. Curr Hypertens Rep 2014;16:450.
[54] Rhoney D, Peacock WF. Intravenous therapy for hypertensive emergencies, part one. Am J Health Syst Pharm 2009;66:1343–52.
[55] James MF. Use of magnesium sulphate in the anesthetic management of phaeochromocytoma: a review of 17 anaesthetics. Br J Anaesth 1989;62:616–23.
[56] Treschan TA, Peters J. The vasopressin system: physiology and clinical strategies. Anesthesiology 2006;105:599–612.
[57] Lord MS, Augoustides JG. Perioperative management of pheochromocytoma: focus on magnesium, clevidipine, and vasopressin. J Cardiothorac Vasc Anesth 2012;26:526–31.
[58] Roth JV. Use of vasopressin bolus and infusion to treat catecholamine-resistant hypotension during pheochromocytoma resection. Anesthesiology 2007;106:883–4.
[59] Holt NF, Haspel KL. Vasopressin: a review of therapeutic applications. J Cardiothorac Vasc Anesth 2010;24:330–47.
[60] Jude EB, Sridhar CB. Prolonged hypoglycaemia following surgical removal of phaeochromocytoma. Postgrad Med J 2000;76:39–40.
[61] Kaya O, Veneman TF, Kruijswijk J, et al. Severe hypoglycemia after resection of adrenal pheochromocytoma: a case report. Eur J Surg 2000;166:974–6.
[62] Chen Y, Hodin RA, Pandolfi C, et al. Hypoglycemia after resection of pheochromocytoma. Surgery 2014;156:1404–8.

FSC
www.fsc.org
MIX
Papier | Fördert gute Waldnutzung
FSC® C083411

Kolibri 360 GmbH
Ferdinand-Jühlke-Straße 7
99095 Erfurt, Deutschland
produktsicherheit@kolibri360.de